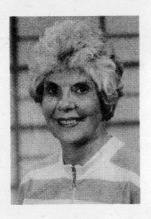

Pat Rowlandson's life-long interest in physical exercise began in the 1930s when she studied ballet in Paris. In 1938 she received her Teaching Diploma from the Women's League of Health and Beauty. For over a decade she represented the WLHB on the Movement and Dance Committee of the Central Council of Physical Recreation, and has been Training Officer for the WLHB since 1982.

In 1980 she began teaching Health in Retirement classes and then EXTEND (Exercise Training for the Elderly and Disabled) courses. She appeared in the Channel 4 programme *Years Ahead* in 1982 and presents the new *Easy Does It!* series.

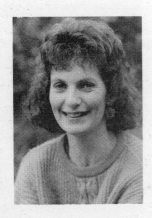

Lesley Hilton is the Associate Producer of the Channel Four/ Yorkshire Television series of *Easy Does It!*. She has worked in television and as a freelance journalist for many years and has a special interest in health matters, particularly in the areas of preventitive and complementary medicine. She lives in West Yorkshire and has three young children.

GW00691579

ACKNOWLEDGEMENTS

Thanks are due to Maggie Raynor for the line drawings; Alan Harbour and Brian Cleasby for the photographs; Zao-Sulle of Image Bank for the cover photograph; the Miriam Stoppard *Health and Beauty Pack* for details on hand massage. Cover design by Studio Gerard.

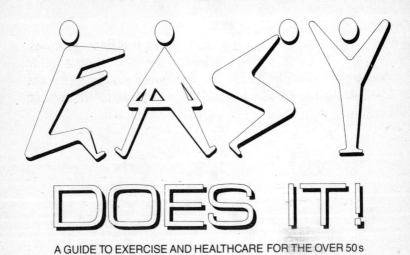

DOES IT!

A GUIDE TO EXERCISE AND HEALTHCARE FOR THE OVER 50s

LESLEY HILTON

Foreword by Pat Rowlandson

In association with Channel Four Television Limited
and Yorkshire Television Limited.

An OPTIMA book

Text word copyright © Yorkshire Television Ltd. 1988
Photographs copyright © Yorkshire Television Ltd. 1988
Illustrations copyright © Maggie Raynor, 1988

First published in 1988 by
Macdonald Optima, a division of
Macdonald & Co. (Publishers) Ltd

A member of Pergamon Publishing Corporation plc

All rights reserved

No part of this publication may be reproduced,
stored in a retrieval system, or transmitted,
in any form or by any means without the prior
permission in writing of the publisher, nor be
otherwise circulated in any form of binding or
cover other than that in which it is published
and without a similar condition including this
condition being imposed on the subsequent
purchaser.

British Library Cataloguing in Publication Data

Hilton, Lesley
    Easy does it.
    1. Old persons. Physical fitness. Exercises
    I. Title   II. Rowlandson, Pat
    613.7′1′0880565
    ISBN 0-356-17524-3

Macdonald & Co. (Publishers) Ltd
3rd Floor
Greater London House
Hampstead Road
London NW1 7QX

Typeset in Century Schoolbook by
Leaper & Gard Ltd, Bristol

Printed and bound in Great Britain by
The Guernsey Press Co Ltd, Guernsey, Channel Islands

CONTENTS

FOREWORD

Fifty years of teaching for the Women's League of Health and Beauty, and more recently with EXTEND (Exercise Training for the Elderly and Disabled) has taught me a great deal about the long-term effects and benefits of well-trained exercise. To see old friends and colleagues now in their 70s and 80s, with one or two even in their 90s, still fit and able to move with grace and comparative ease, retaining a good degree of independence, is a heartening and satisfying experience.

Exercise alone is not a magic formula, but it can help to prevent and alleviate some of the stressful conditions encountered in our senior years. Add a sensible diet, some general care and mental stimulus, and we have a good recipe for a long and happy retirement. And even if fate treats us harshly and we succumb to ill health, a positive attitude towards health can often help us to recover.

There is a large range of activities for you to choose from which you will find recommended in this book — dancing, swimming, walking, even singing. And you will find some tips which could prove useful in your leisure years.

To join some form of movement class of your own choosing is a great way not only to benefit from the exercise but also to meet new friends and to participate in some of the social activities that are offered. It is particularly beneficial to have someone — a group leader or teacher — to monitor your progress. They will help and encourage you, and you will be able to see how other class members are progressing.

If joining a class is not practical for you, then a regular exercise routine at home is certainly worth considering, providing that your health will allow it. If you are not certain, do get medical advice. A few exercises each day — perhaps four or five minutes to start with, gradually increasing to ten or fifteen — is more beneficial than a long tiring session once a week. Perhaps you have a friend who would like to join you; working out the exercises together could be fun.

Whatever you decide is best, I do hope that you are able to participate in some form of exercise. It is never too late to try, and if you derive the same pleasure and benefits from it as I and many others have, it will be well worth while.

Pat Rowlandson

1
INTRODUCTION

WHY EXERCISE?

Regular gentle exercise can help prevent many of the aches and pains we get as we grow older. It can also be fun and help you get more out of life. Exercise helps you sleep better, can relieve depression, and increases the elasticity of your skin, so helping you to look younger.

Still not convinced? Well, exercise can help to prevent heart disease and high blood pressure, keep your weight down, prevent your muscles from weakening, and keep your joints flexible. Best of all, it can improve your general health and increase your resistance to illness and infection.

As we grow older changes occur in our bodies. Joints become stiffer and perhaps arthritic or rheumatic. We can relieve this by doing exercises to keep them mobile and to strengthen the muscles.

Circulation may become sluggish. Regular exercise will tone it up and keep you warm in the winter.

Your balance may worsen. Achieving a better posture will help to counteract this. Your self-confidence may start to go. Learning to sit and stand tall can help here.

And last but not least, exercise can be great fun, adding to both your physical and mental alertness and relaxation. It can help put those worries into their right perspective. And it can make you a lot of new friends.

> Exercise has helped in a lot of ways, with my breathing. It's hard to explain really, but I feel so much better. I haven't felt like this for years.
>
> *Cathy*, 67.

> I think that exercising will help to keep your muscles supple — you won't be inclined to stiffen up the same. I think that it's so easy when you are older to sit around instead of keeping active.
>
> *May,* 70.

WHERE CAN YOU EXERCISE?

The exercises shown in the book (and the television series) will help to keep you supple if you practise them regularly at home (every day if you can).

If you feel more adventurous, though, you could join an exercise class — there is bound to be one near you. Don't feel that you have to look for a class that is specially for older people. Any good exercise teacher will be able to incorporate you into a mixed-age-group class. But make sure that the teacher has proper qualifications to teach exercise.

Ask at your local library, sports centre or council offices for a list of what's available in your area. Many places have special activities for pensioners now, with centres putting on special programmes on certain days of the week.

If you hear of an activity which you would like to do but which isn't available near you, ask if it can be provided. We filmed an aquatic keep-fit class near Sheffield, and many people have subsequently said they would like to go to one. There aren't many classes like that around, but if something like that takes your fancy, ask for it.

AM I HEALTHY ENOUGH?

Most people can start exercising straight away, but if you have any of the following problems you should ask your doctor which is the best form of exercise for you:

- Chest pains, high blood pressure, heart disease
- Chest trouble such as asthma or bronchitis
- Slipped disc or back problems

- Arthritis, joint pains
- Diabetes
- Recently had a serious illness or an operation

Even if you are disabled you can still exercise. In fact, it is very important that you keep as many of your muscles working as possible. If you can't move your legs, perhaps someone else could help move them for you. And if you are lying in bed you can still exercise your arms and hands, or do the relaxation exercises.

MAKE YOURSELF COMFORTABLE

When you exercise you need to wear something loose and comfortable. Make sure you have enough space to move freely. And don't exercise on a full stomach — wait until about an hour after a meal.

For the sitting exercises you need to make sure that the chair you are using is sturdy. It is better if it has no arms. You can use the same chair to give you support if you need it during the standing exercises.

All the exercises we show are gentle, but it is still a good idea to have a little warm-up before you start. Warm muscles are less likely to get injured. So rub your hands up and down your legs and arms. Shake your hands. Bounce on the spot a few times. That should loosen you up ready to start exercising.

In the television programmes we developed our exercise routines to a piece of music. You might find that doing an exercise to a favourite song is more fun and helps you keep to a rhythm more easily than doing it in silence. But never let the music force the pace for you — after the exercise you should feel pleasantly stretched and warm, not uncomfortably breathless or in anyway distressed.

> I feel much fitter, more supple. I don't puff as much and I like the activity of it. Where I live it's very steep and I can get up and down the path without panting a lot easier now than I used to be able to do. I really feel the benefit.
> *Nancy*, 71.

HEALTHY LIVING AND EATING

When you are retired you have more time to look after yourself, so make the most of it. You should have regular health checks. Ask your doctor to check your blood pressure every few months. He/she can also test your blood to see what your cholesterol level is and then advise you on any changes you need to make to your diet to cut down your risk of heart disease.

Women should also have cervical smear tests — see your GP for that or perhaps go to a well-woman clinic. Even if you don't have sex any more you may still be at risk from developing cancer of the cervix.

It is important that you eat well — quality is more important than quantity now. Eat more poultry and fish, and cut down on red meat, sugar and dairy products. Make sure you get plenty of fibre, from foods like whole-meal bread, fresh fruit and vegetables.

Perhaps you don't have much of an appetite any more, especially if you have lost your sense of taste or smell. But don't make the mistake of over-salting your food to compensate — too much salt is bad for you. Try adding herbs or garlic to get more flavour.

If you have difficulty in swallowing or chewing your food, perhaps because you have to wear dentures, make sure that you always have a drink with your meal. Or have gravy or a sauce to make the food more moist.

If you find it a chore to cook for just yourself why don't you get together with a friend and share your meals? Take it in turns to cook. Or cook in batches so you don't have to make a meal every day.

Here are several guidelines you could follow to give yourself a healthier diet.

I've always been interested in exercise, and over the past few years I've tried to keep myself active in one form or another. I think coming to keep-fit class is great. As you get older I think you should be looking to look after yourself more.

Tom, 65.

- Buy wholemeal bread and use wholemeal flour in your baking. Use wholemeal pasta and cereals and brown rice.
- Eat lots of fresh fruit and vegetables, salads and potatoes.
- Grill food instead of frying it.
- Cut down on sweets, cakes, biscuits and puddings. Have a piece of fresh fruit, some unsalted nuts or a plain yogurt instead.
- Eat more fish. Doctors believe that the Japanese rarely suffer from heart disease because they eat a lot of oily fish such as herring and mackerel. Fish oil lowers the cholesterol level in the blood and reduces the risk of clots forming in the blood vessels and blocking them.
- Cut down on the amount of fat you eat. Switch to skimmed or semi-skimmed milk and dairy products and use a margarine high in polyunsaturated fats instead of butter. Use low-fat cheese such as Edam.
- Sugar doesn't provide you with anything except empty calories, and there is evidence that it might make you more prone to infections. Try to cut it out of your diet. Make sure you look down the list of ingredients on packaged foods to see if they contain sugar. Don't forget that sucrose, glucose, dextrose, maltose and fructose are all forms of sugar.
- Don't drink too much coffee. Researchers have found that five or more cups a day could cause heart disease. (Heart disease is responsible for one in three deaths among people over the age of 45, and is six times more common in men than women.)

Don't get stuck in a rut — try to keep an element of choice and flexibility in your life. And do try to get out for a little fresh air every day. When you live on your own or are a little unsteady on your feet it can become a major effort to get out of the house. But you should try. Or sit by an open window every day and do some deep breathing. Recent research has shown that sunlight can actually help prevent depression in some people, so get out in it if you can.

AND FINALLY

Finally, remember that exercise isn't just about keeping your body fit. It's about having fun and feeling good about yourself too. And age is no barrier to enjoyment. Try not to get depressed by the things you can't do any more and think positively about what you can do.

USEFUL INFORMATION

The following addresses may be useful if you want to make your life healthier.

The Sports Council
16 Upper Woburn Place
London WC1H 0QP
01-388 1277
They have leaflets for older people giving advice on various sports and can give you the address of the governing body of any specific sport you are interested in. They also have regional offices.

Citizens Advice Bureaux
There are offices all over the country (see local phone book) and they provide information on what is available locally.
If you don't have a local office write to:
National Association of Citizens Advice Bureaux
115–123 Pentonville Road
London N1 9LZ
01-833 2181

Action on Smoking and Health (ASH)
5–11 Mortimer Street
London W1N 7RN
01-637 9843
Will give advice on how to stop smoking and how to campaign for smoke-free zones.

Alcohol Concern
305 Gray's Inn Road
London WC1X 8QF
01-883 3471
Have over 40 local advice centres where you can get advice
and support to cut down on alcohol.

Keep Fit Association
16 Upper Woburn Place
London WC1H 0QC
01-387 4349
Will give details of classes run by KFA qualified teachers.

Age Concern have information and give advice on all
matters of concern to older people. They also run local
groups and send out fact sheets.

Age Concern England
60 Pitcairn Road
Mitcham
Surrey CR4 3LL
01-640 5431

Age Concern Northern Ireland
128 Great Victoria Street
Belfast BT2 7BG
0232 245729

Age Concern Scotland
33 Castle Street
Edinburgh EH2 3DN
031-225 5000

Age Concern Wales
1 Park Grove
Cardiff CF1 3BJ
0222 371821/371566

British Diabetic Association
10 Queen Anne Street
London W1M 0BD
01-323 1531

Health Education Authority
78 New Oxford Street
London WC1A 1AH
01-631 0903
Has information on all aspects of health, nutrition and exercise. (See also your local Health Education Unit in your phonebook under your local district health authority.

Look After Yourself! These are courses run locally to show you how to live more healthily whatever age you are.
Contact:
Project Centre
Christchurch College
Canterbury
Kent CT1 1QU
0227 455564

Pre-Retirement Association
19 Undine Street
London SW17 8PP
A government backed body responsible for preparing people for retirement.

Pensioners Link (London only)
17 Balfe Street
London N1 9EB

The Prime of Your Life, Miriam Stoppard, Penguin Books, £5.95

Second Bite of the Cherry: Eating for Health and Pleasure in the Middle Years, Alan Stewart and Margaret Jackson, Macdonald Optima, £5.99

Know Your Medicines, Dr Pat Blair, from Age Concern, £3.75

Keeping Warm on a Pension, London Energy and Employment Network, 99 Midland Road, London NW1 2AH, 50p

Enjoy Sex in the Middle Years, Dr Christine E Sandford, Macdonald Optima/Positive Health Guides, £4.99

Diabetes Beyond 40, Dr Rowan Hillson, Macdonald Optima/Positive Health Guides, £5.99

When I started classes I was very stiff. I couldn't bend, I couldn't do this, I couldn't do that, I couldn't get my arm up. Now I can and it's been the best thing that could have happened to me. I really enjoy every minute. And when I saw the specialist in the hospital, he said I'd done tremendously well and it would be coming to the class that's done it. It really has helped me an awful lot.

Jean, 69.

Coming to the class has helped me with my gardening. I lost my husband, which left me with a big garden, and all this exercise helps me with the digging and dragging and pulling about. I enjoy it very much indeed and I've met a lot of people. It gives you some time out, whereas you'd be lost in your own home.

Mabel, 64.

2
HOW TO USE THIS BOOK

The exercises in this book are designed with different abilities in mind. Retirement onwards covers a very wide age range and as we grow older changes occur in our bodies and in our general make-up, so don't press yourself too hard.

Towards the end of each chapter there are three or four different exercises. The easiest ones come first. Try each slowly and carefully. If you feel breathless or in any discomfort, don't persist. In a class, the teacher can advise you. On your own, 'easy does it'.

Once each movement is understood and mastered, try the next. If you are fit and agile try the whole section, which should add up to a short 1-minute work-out. This will give you variety, and provide a minor stamina test.

If you enjoy moving to music, try working to some of your favourite tunes, but don't allow the music to dictate an unreasonable speed.

When exercising clothing should be comfortable, not too tight or too warm — a leisure suit, or trousers and top, are suitable. The room should be warm enough but well ventilated. Allow plenty of space — furniture, etc., well out of reach. And never exercise immediately after a big meal. As a preliminary to any exercising, the following tips are useful.

CHAIR EXERCISES

Chair exercises allow plenty of movement with the weight off your feet and legs. The chair needs to be very stable and without arms if possible, with a fairly firm seat and back to support you.

Sitting tall

Lower your back well into the chair, with your upper legs completely supported and your feet slightly apart. Your feet should be flat on the floor, your shoulders directly over the hips, arms down to your sides, the crown of your head pushed towards the ceiling.

STANDING EXERCISES

Standing exercises (if you can manage them) will help to strengthen your feet and legs. Your chair should be high enough for you to stand behind it and place your hands comfortably on the back — this will assist your balance.

Standing tall

Your feet should be comfortably straight and slightly apart, with your legs as straight as possible. Your trunk, head and arms should be as in the sitting position, top of the head (not your chin) pushed towards the ceiling.

LYING EXERCISES

Some lying exercises will be described later in the book. These provide a particularly good position in which to practise relaxation. You can either use a bed, preferably a firm one, or a rug on the floor if you can manage it.

WARMING UP

This is a warm-up and general exercise routine which you could easily practise every day.

Arms

- Rub your arms alternately, first one then the other.

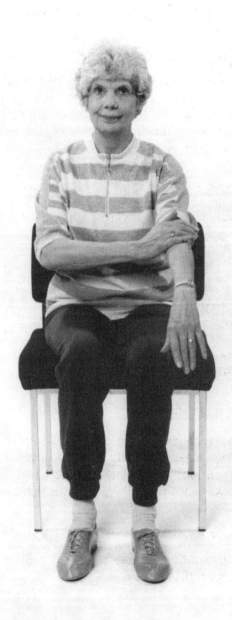

- Bend your arms so that your hands touch the front of your shoulders.

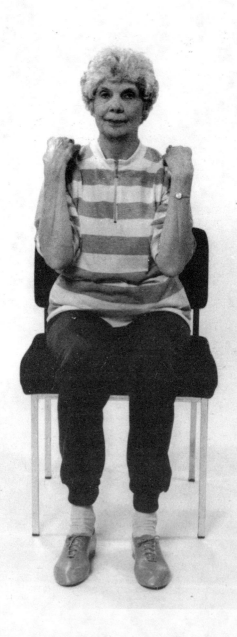

- Then stretch out your arms straight in front of you at shoulder level, and bend them back again as before.

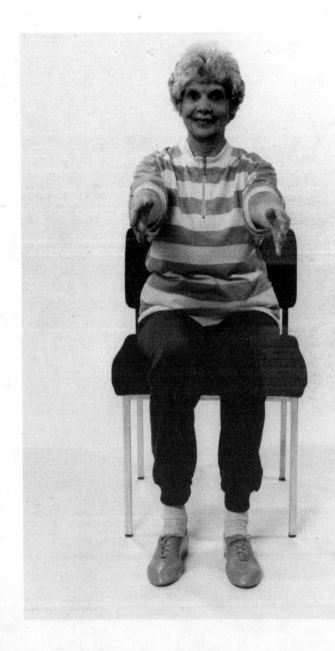

- Bend your arms so your hands are on your shoulders again, then stretch them out sideways at shoulder level. Bend your arms back to the original position again.

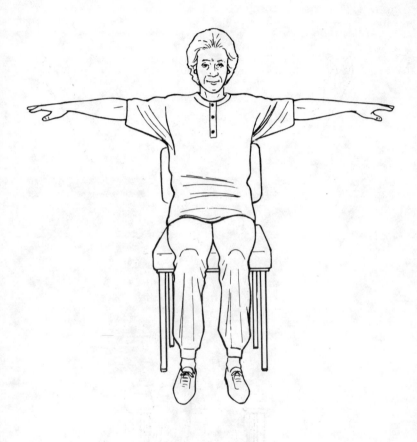

I feel better in every way — muscles, everything. And then at the end of the day I do relax because the muscles have been into play and you just feel as though you want to relax.

Annie, 62.

- Put your hands on your shoulders, then straighten your arms, raising them upwards slightly. Return your hands to your shoulders, then put your arms down by your side.

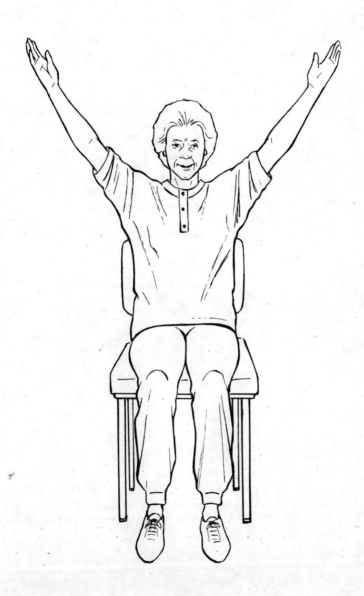

Legs

- Rub your thighs and rub gently over your knee joint, massaging as far down the leg as possible. Then sit up.

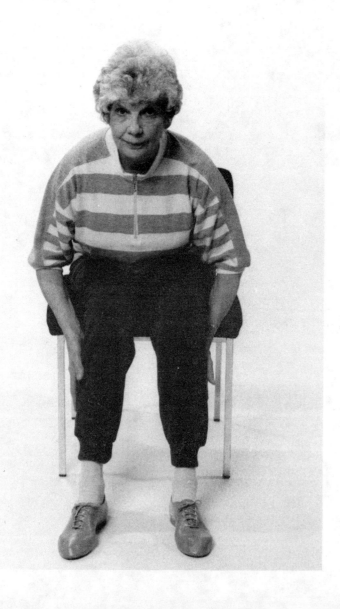

- To test the range of movement in your legs, support one leg with both hands under the thigh and with your knee bent.

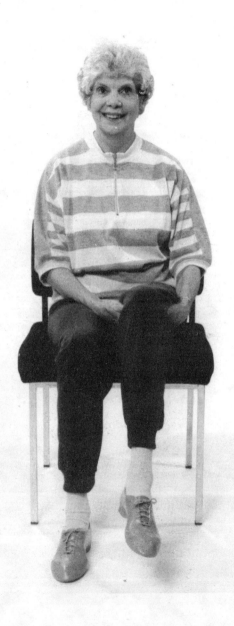

- Then lift your leg and stretch it forwards as far as it is comfortable.

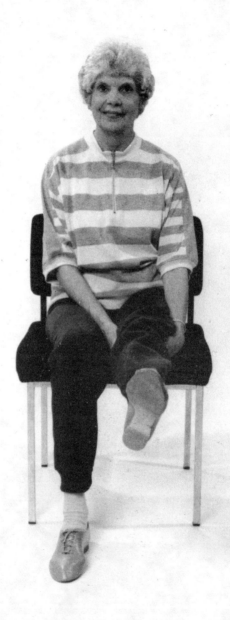

- Do 16 'walks' on the spot.

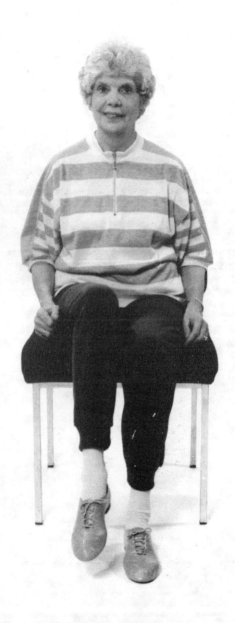

- Slowly lift each leg a little way off the chair, with the knee bent. Tap the thigh with the opposite hand. Do this six times in all.

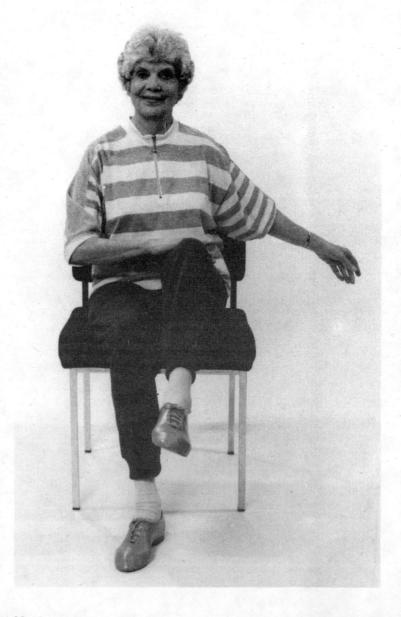

Trunk

- Place your feet apart firmly on the floor.
- Clap your hands to the right, then swing round and clap your hands to the left.

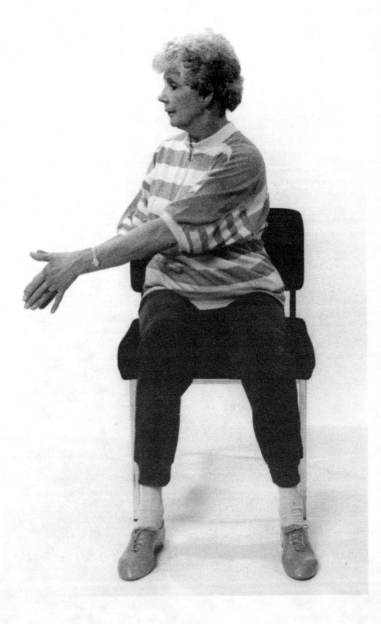

- Tap the top of your thighs and stretch forward to clap your hands in front of you.

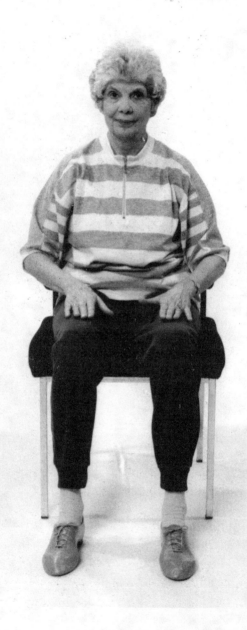

- Repeat these movements up to four times, allowing the trunk of your body to follow your arm movements.

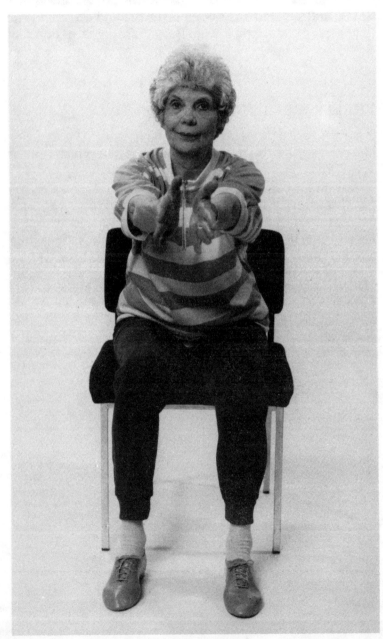

WARMING-UP TO MUSIC

Once you have carried out this warm-up routine a few times, find some bright marching music and see if you can fit the work-out to the music. But don't rush it — don't let the music impose an uncomfortable rhythm on the exercises.

THE USEFUL INFORMATION SECTION

You will see at the end of most chapters that there is a section entitled 'Useful information'. This is just what it says it is.

Any organisation that is mentioned in a chapter will have its full address and, where possible, telephone number listed in this section. We have also listed a few books in some cases, as well as other organisations that will be able to help in specific circumstances. These sections are therefore designed to give you as much back-up information as possible.

3
BREATHING

There's more to breathing than just getting air into and out of your lungs. Learning to breathe better can give you more energy and lift your spirits too.

Deep breathing also helps your body to get rid of the poisons that build up in us all. The extra oxygen increases your powers of concentration and makes your circulation work better.

DO YOU BREATHE BADLY?

Most of us take breathing for granted until we have trouble with it. But in fact a lot of us breathe too shallowly most of the time, which means we are not getting the benefits that the extra oxygen can give us.

If you breathe only in your upper chest you get tired more quickly, and can get pains in your chest, sometimes so bad that you think you are about to have a heart attack. Shallow breathing may cause palpitations, and they may even cause panic attacks. And if you suffer from asthma you make an attack more likely by not breathing correctly.

Stress can be a major cause of breathing too fast and too lightly. Learn to relax and take slow, regular breaths that fill the whole chest. Many cardiac units in hospitals are now starting to teach deep breathing to their patients to help them to relax.

Well I was retired. I've always been interested in music and it is very enjoyable singing together. We have a laugh and a bit of fun — it's not too serious.

Dick, 70.

OVERBREATHING

Overbreathing in your upper chest can make you feel giddy and faint. If this happens to you, try taking a few breaths into a paper bag or your cupped hands. Relax your tongue to the bottom of your mouth — this will also relax your throat.

Relaxing your tongue like this and taking deep, regular breaths will help you overcome a panic attack too. Always try to breathe in through your nose and not through your mouth.

GOOD BREATHING

It is important that you learn the habit of breathing correctly, and any exercise that helps is a good idea — cycling, walking and swimming are all excellent for getting extra air into your lungs.

Of course, it's even better if you can make sure that the air is fresh and clean too. But even if you live in a city, try to get out for a walk every day. Or sit by an open window and do some deep breathing if you are housebound.

If you find it hard to concentrate on breathing exercises, try singing or whistling to yourself. You are then controlling your breath without really noticing. Humming is another good thing to do, as the vibrations help to massage the air passages. Try humming one note for as long as you can, or humming a tune without pausing for breath (you'll have to take a deep breath at the end). Humming, singing and whistling are all good tension relievers too.

IMPROVING YOUR BREATHING

If you suffer from asthma, bronchitis or breathlessness you should not smoke, neither should you spend a lot of time in the company of others who do smoke. Contact ASH if you want to give up.

Having an ioniser in the room can help you to breath better. So can keeping the room warm (but not stuffy), well-ventilated and humidified.

Swimming is a good exercise for asthmatics as it strengthens the lungs and develops the ribcage. Learning a relaxation technique can also help you as it calms you down and teaches you how to breathe deeply. The Alexander Technique, by improving your posture, helps with breathing too.

If you suffer from chronic catarrh cut down on milk, dairy products and sugar in your diet. Increase the amount of fresh fruit and vegetables that you eat, and try to have onions and garlic often, as these are said to help reduce mucus. You could also try taking 500 mg vitamin C pills three times a day, especially in the winter.

If you have a cold and can't breathe properly when you lie down to sleep, prop yourself up into a more upright position with pillows, and take deep slow breaths. Once you feel better or your cold has gone, though, don't go on sleeping in that position because it is bad for your back.

SINGING AND MUSIC-MAKING

If you like the idea of singing and would like to take it more seriously, then why not join a choir? There are thousands of them all over the country. Many are just groups of people who get together to sing just for the sheer joy of it. They are not all attached to churches, and groups like the University of the Third Age have local choir groups around the country.

Playing a wind instrument will help you to develop good breathing habits, too. If you used to play one and haven't done so for years, perhaps you could take it up again.

BEFORE YOU START

Breathing exercises can be done sitting, lying or standing. Build up to deep breathing gradually, otherwise you could get dizzy. And before you start the breathing exercises take a small breath in and then exhale fully (and make sure you always exhale fully after a deep intake of breath).

Breathe in for two counts and out for two at a moderate

> I spent 40 years down the pit and I suffered from lack of breath and wheezing in the morning. Coming to the choir and learning to breathe properly has really helped me and I hope it continues to do so for many years to come.
>
> *Bob*, 67.

speed. Then increase to four counts in and four counts out. (If you want to do this to music, a moderate waltz fits nicely.) Breathe in for two counts and out for six to make sure that you fully exhale. Keep the breathing even and regular.

As you breathe in, allow your tummy muscles to relax. You will then be able to breathe right down to your lowest ribs. If you place your hands on the ribcage you can feel the movement as it fills with air.

Now try the illustrated exercises, bringing in the arm movements.

DEEP BREATHING

This will help your poise and improve your posture, as well as calming and relaxing you.

Always breathe in through the nose, and gradually increase to a deeper breath until you reach your comfortable maximum — do not strain. Put your hands on your ribcage and feel it expand as you breathe in. Fill all the space you can find in your lungs before gently exhaling. And always keep the tummy muscles relaxed.

- Sit upright, but not rigid, in a chair.
- Place your hands lightly towards the front of the ribcage. The arms and shoulders should be relaxed.
- Breathe in for two counts and out for two counts.
- Do this three times, then go back to your normal breathing.

If you feel dizzy you are over-inhaling — breathe in in a more relaxed style, and don't force it.

A slow waltz will provide the right sort of timing for this breathing.

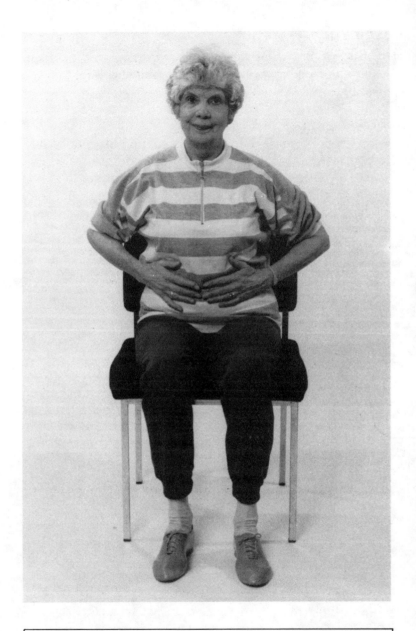

When I'm walking uphill I get a touch of angina ... and that's not very nice. But I find that doing the breathing exercises helps.

Catherine, 70.

Using the arms

- Repeat your deep breathing exercise, but lift your arms from your sides up to shoulder level as you inhale.

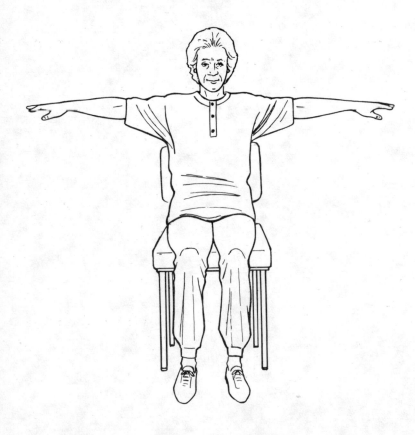

When I started at first I found that I was short of breath, I just couldn't manage the exercises without running out of puff. But you acclimatise after a week or two and you find that you've got much more energy than you thought you had; whereas if you sit at home, then the less you do the less you want to do.

Ernest, 66.

- Then bring them down to your sides again as you exhale.
- Repeat, lifting your arms a little higher.

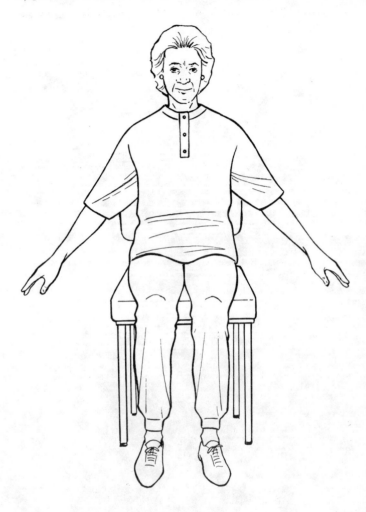

I enjoy the voice exercises, the breathing exercises, and I find it helps me when I have to go uphill. And I so enjoy coming because I love the singing and I love the company. I think everybody who is elderly should have an interest. I think it helps to keep you going.

Edith, 69.

- Repeat, lifting your arms as high as possible without straining.

Try not to shrug your shoulders as you move your arms.

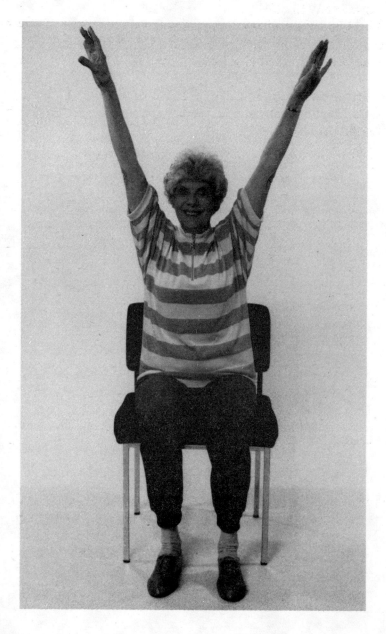

USEFUL INFORMATION

University of the Third Age
6 Parkside Gardens
London SW19 5EY
The University of the Third Age have local choir groups around the country. If you want a list, write, enclosing a stamped addressed envelope

Action on Smoking and Health (ASH)
5–11 Mortimer Street
London W1N 7RN
01-637 9843

Chest, Heart and Stroke Association
Tavistock House North
Tavistock Square
London WC1H 9JE
01-387 3012

Society of Alexander Technique Teachers
18 Lansdowne Road
London W11
01-272 7222

Alexander Technique, Chris Stevens, Macdonald Optima, £3.95

Kick It! Stop Smoking in 5 days, Judy Perlmutter, Thorsons, £1.99

Ionisers are known to be particularly helpful to people with respiratory problems, and they help to reduce air pollution. For further information and mail order details, please contact:

Mountain Breeze Air Ionisers
Peel House
Peel Road
Skelmersdale
Lancashire WN8 9PT
0695 21155

4
RELAXATION

These days we are always being told to relax. Unfortunately stress and tension seem to be part and parcel of life when you are bringing up a family or holding down a job. That tension doesn't always go away when you retire or your family grows up — worries about money or health can still loom large.

STRESS AND TENSION

Tension shows itself in various ways. You may be tired and irritable all the time for no apparent reason. You may have trouble sleeping. You may grind your teeth or frown a lot.

Headaches and pains in the chest can all be the results of being tense all the time and can lead in time to heart attacks. Continual clenching and unclenching of the hands is another tell-tale sign that you are not relaxed. Or your shoulders might be hunched up.

EXERCISE AND RELAX

If you recognise these signs in yourself you must learn to relax. There are basically two ways of doing this.

One is to be out and have fun! Go dancing, go to an exercise class or join a walking club.

Researchers have found that there is a link between exercise and the chemicals in our brains that can cause depression. Exercise can actually lift our spirits and make us feel happier by changing those chemicals. And of course, exercise is also relieving muscle tension at the same time.

It can be hard to think that you can exercise if you are fairly immobile. But it is very good for you to exercise the parts of your body that you can still move and, as we found during our filming, even very frail pensioners in a day-care centre looked forward to their weekly exercise class.

If you attend a day-care centre or live in a residential home, why don't you ask the person in charge if they would arrange an exercise session on a regular basis. Some homes have visiting keep-fit and yoga teachers every week, and they all have great fun.

RELAXATION AND YOGA

The other way to relax is less energetic.

Learn a relaxation technique, or listen to relaxing music. Find out about aromatherapy — different essential oils can have a relaxing effect. A few drops of lavender, chamomile or orange-blossom oil in your bath might make all the difference.

If you live in rooms that are decorated in bright colours such as red or orange, they might be over-stimulating you. Pale blues and greens are thought to be the most soothing colours to surround yourself with.

Taking up an activity such as t'ai chi or yoga can also be very helpful. Yoga is a method of doing gentle exercises that not only stretches your muscles and tones your body, but also calms your mind and relaxes you. It is best to go to a class with a qualified yoga teacher to learn the basic routines, but once you have learned them you can do yoga at home on your own.

There are many yoga classes available now all round the country — ask at your local library or leisure centre. Or you could write to the British Wheel of Yoga or one of the other yoga organisations and get a list of qualified yoga teachers from them.

Yoga, and in fact many other forms of exercise, teaches you how to reach out and stretch.

T'AI CHI

Both yoga and t'ai chi have been around for thousands of years, but it is only recently that they have become popular in the West. Yoga is comparatively well known now, but you may not have heard of t'ai chi.

T'ai chi is an ancient Chinese system of exercises. It involves very slow and balanced movements, and is well suited to the not-so-young. As well as keeping you flexible and supple, it brings your body into balance and makes you more aware and relaxed within yourself.

As with yoga, many adult education centres and leisure centres now give t'ai chi classes — see if any are available in your area.

RELAXING AT BEDTIME

A lot of people find it harder to get to sleep at night as they get older. One reason for this is simply that we actually need less sleep at this stage in our life, especially if you are taking one or more naps during the day. Accept it and you won't lie in bed worrying that you are not getting enough sleep.

Go to bed a bit later than you are used to and don't go to bed at all until you actually feel tired. Have a milky drink or a light snack before bed — being hungry can keep you awake. Malted milk drinks are good, or a bowl of cereal — there seems to be something in the combination of milk and cereal that induces sleep.

Establishing a bedtime routine can also be helpful. Have a warm bath before you try to sleep. Read in bed if you find that helps. Not too exciting a book though — that will only keep you awake.

A bedtime relaxation
Try this relaxation technique once you are in bed.

- Lie on your back with a pillow under your head.
- Tighten the muscles of the right arm to three slow counts and relax to four counts.

- Repeat with the left arm.
- Repeat with both arms. Include the shoulders, neck and facial muscles (screw up your face) to the count of three, and relax.
- Repeat using the right leg, then the left leg, to the count of three, and then relax.
- Do the same thing once more using both legs together, tightening your tummy muscles as well. Relax and rest for a moment.
- Finally, tense all your limbs and your body to a count of three, as before, then relax. Repeat this three times.

WORKING ON THE BLADDER

While we are on the subject of tensing and relaxing muscles, women may find it useful to learn how to strengthen the muscles which control the bladder.

All you need to do is slowly tighten the muscles around that area, hold it for a second or two and then relax. Practise several times a day.

When you are doing it properly you should be able to stop the flow of urine at will when you are spending a penny.

PREVENTING LEG CRAMPS

If you get cramps in your legs at night try gently stretching the cramped muscle against the contraction and rub the affected area to relieve the pain. Breathe slowly and deeply.

Keeping your feet and legs warm by wearing bedsocks sometimes helps prevent cramp. Alternatively, some people swear by a good old-fashioned mustard bath. It perks up the circulation and may help to keep cramps at bay. Put one tablespoonful of mustard powder in enough water to cover the feet. Bathe the feet for three minutes and splash the calves as well. Do this three times a week.

Taking extra vitamin E and calcium can also help — ask your doctor, or buy them at a chemists or health-food store.

RELAX AND HAVE FUN

This movement can be used to stretch, to give your body a swing and to relax it. It is not a formal exercise, so feel free to vary it as you want. It should be fun.

- Sit in a chair with a light headscarf or square in the right hand.
- Raise the right hand to shoulder level, sweeping the headscarf upwards.
- Gently swing your arm up and circle the scarf over your head, passing it to the other hand.

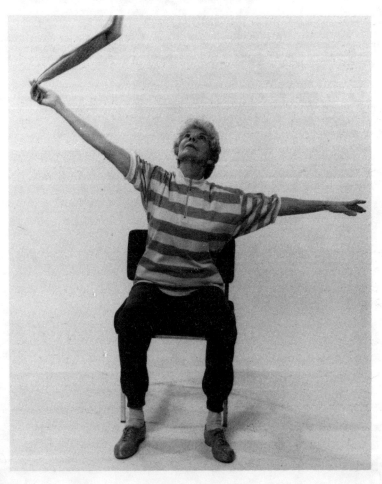

- Swing the other arm down.
- Reverse the movement.

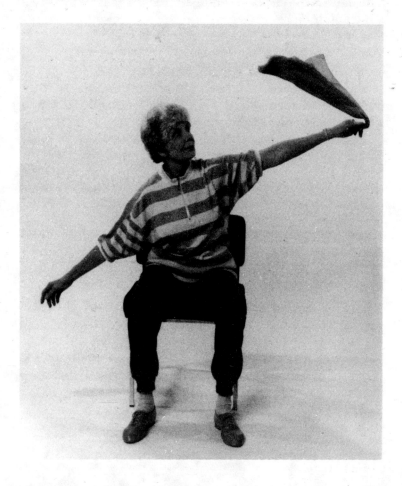

You should be able to achieve a combination of swings and circles, stretching a variety of muscles and improving the movement of all the arm and shoulder joints.

> I enjoy singing because I think it makes you feel more cheerful.
>
> *Margaret,* 68.

USEFUL INFORMATION

The British Wheel of Yoga
1 Hamilton Place
Sleaford
Lincs
0529 306851
The British Wheel of Yoga have the largest list of registered yoga teachers in the UK, and will probably be able to advise you of one running classes near you.

Yoga for Health Foundation
Ickwell Bury
Biggleswade
Bedfordshire SG18 9EF
076 727 271
The Yoga for Health Foundation specialises in remedial, therapeutic and preventative yoga, and you might well find that their style of yoga is more suited to you.

The British School of Yoga
24 Osney Crescent
Paignton
Devon TQ4 5EY
0803 552090

Iyengar Yoga Institute
223A Randolph Avenue
London W9 1NL
01-624 3080

Sivananda Yoga Centre
50 Chepstow Villas
London W11
01-229 7970

Scottish Yoga Association
4 Afton Place
Edinburgh EH5 3RB

British T'ai Chi Ch'uan Association
7 Upper Wimpole Street
London W1M 7TD
01-933 8444

Relaxation for Living
29 Burwood Park Road
Walton-on-Thames
Surrey KT12 5LH
This is a charity which promotes relaxation as a means of coping with stress and strain. Send a stamped addressed envelope for information.

Stress and Relaxation, Jane Madders, Macdonald Optima/Positive Health Guides, £4.99

Keep Moving — Keep Young, Margaret Graham, Unwin Hyman, £6.95

Practical Aromatherapy, Shirley Price, Thorsons, £4.99

5
BALANCE

If you find it hard to keep your balance, you don't move around so much, and then you start to stiffen up ... which makes it even harder to get around. So it is worth working on your balancing act.

To keep your balance you need to have good coordination, and regular exercise can help improve this. Activities which are especially good for improving your balance are yoga, dance, t'ai chi and fencing. (And when you get really good you could even learn to roller-skate!)

POSTURE AND CONFIDENCE

To keep your balance your posture needs to be good (see the next chapter, on posture). Each of your weight-bearing joints (feet, knees, hips, spine) need to be correctly positioned, one over the other, with your head held upright and eyes looking straight ahead. Then your centre of gravity will be in the right place.

But being able to keep your balance isn't just a question of having all your joints in the right place. Like so many other things, it also depends on your confidence in your own ability. If you have already had a bad fall it will probably have shaken your self-confidence and you will have to work at getting it back again. Standing tall and feeling confident is the key to success.

> Knowing that some movement has to be done, and then converting that into movement of the arm and leg isn't something that I've been used to doing. I've had a desk job all my life and doing something active is great fun, yes.
>
> *Harold,* 66.

> I think fencing's helped my overall fitness. You're on your feet and you have to keep your balance. And you're using muscles you don't use in other exercises.
>
> *Jean*, 60.
>
> I took up fencing because I wanted something which I thought was different, and would be easy, you know, not too strenuous. But I found out it was pretty strenuous exercise. You use the calf muscles, your thigh muscles and of course your arm muscles. And believe me, after a while of doing it you can feel those muscles.
>
> Mary, 60.

REASONS FOR BAD BALANCE

There are some physical reasons why you may find it hard to keep your balance. If there is a problem with your eyes you should get them checked regularly. Your eyesight changes over the years and if you wear glasses they may need changing.

Or an ear infection can throw you off balance — you may not even have earache to warn you about it. If your balance suddenly worsens, see your doctor and ask for your ears to be checked.

Ménière's disease, which is caused by an increase in the pressure of the fluids in the inner ear, can cause you to have giddy spells. If your doctor diagnoses this you may find that reducing the amount of salt and caffeine in your diet may help you. For more information on Ménière's disease write to the Ménière's Society.

If you are regularly taking tranquillisers or sleeping pills they may be making you feel a little unsteady on your feet during the day. Doctors issue 24 million prescriptions each year for these sorts of drugs and it is believed that up to a third of those who become addicted to them are over the age of 55. If you are on these drugs and feel they may be affecting your balance, ask your doctor if you can reduce the dose or if you really need them at all.

If you need extra help to come off them contact Tranx (UK) Ltd.

DON'T TAKE RISKS

One of the biggest causes of accidents among older people is probably from falls, many of them caused by falling off a chair while trying to reach something on a high shelf.

Be sensible. Don't stand on wobbly stools or chairs. Invest in a good pair of steps with a handrail and a platform at the top. Don't keep things on high shelves. Ask for help when reaching for things. Don't even try to take the curtains down by yourself if you are at all unsteady on your feet.

And don't climb up on something at all if you are feeling hungry — you are more likely to feel faint.

EXERCISES TO IMPROVE BALANCE

A simple exercise
This is a good exercise to help your balance.

- Hold on to the back of a steady chair or table (when you get more confident you can do the exercise without support).
- Just raise your heels up so you are standing on your toes and then lower them again.
  Do this several times.
- This is also a good strengthening exercise for your calf muscles, but don't repeat it too often without a rest or they will get over-tired.

A variation
Use a chair if necessary. Stand behind it or to one side, with your feet comfortably apart and pointing straight ahead.

Well I like fencing because it's a different sport. It's something different to do. And it's something that I'd never done before.

Daisy, 66.

- Keeping a good erect position, bend your knees.
- Straighten your knees.
- Rise on to the ball of each foot, then place the heels back on the floor.

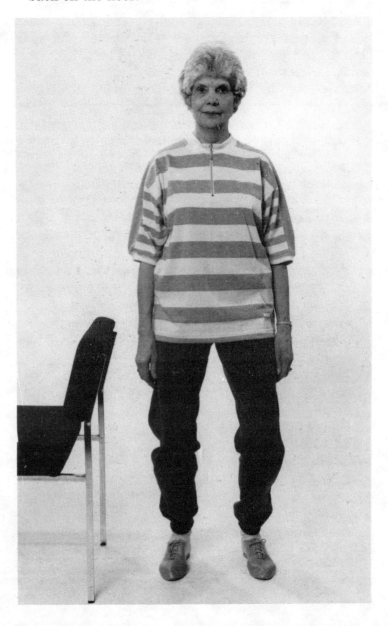

- Do this three times.

You can test your balance by letting go of the chair-back while you are up on the balls of your feet.

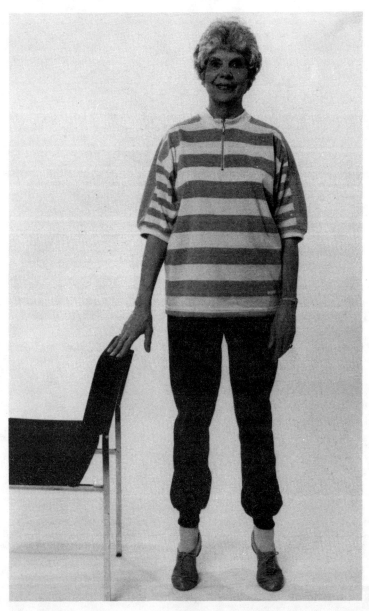

Swaying

- Take up a standing position with the feet apart.
- Bend both knees.

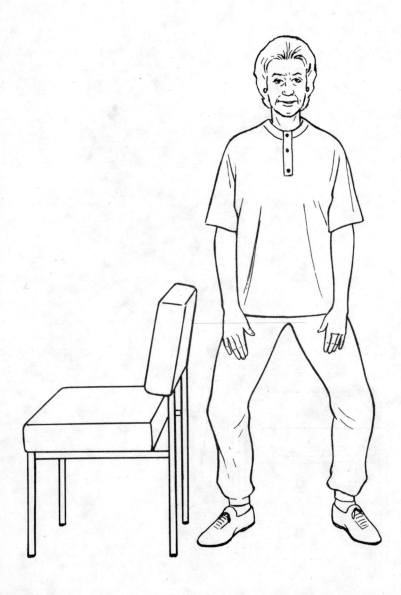

- Transfer your weight on to your right foot, straightening your legs.
- Repeat in the other direction, finishing with your weight on the left foot.
- Do four complete sways, swaying from leg to leg.

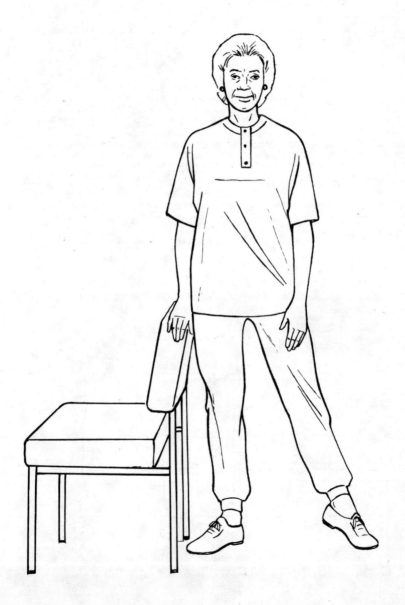

Lunge

- From a standing position with your legs apart, bend your right knee over your right foot, extending your right arm. Keep your left leg straight.

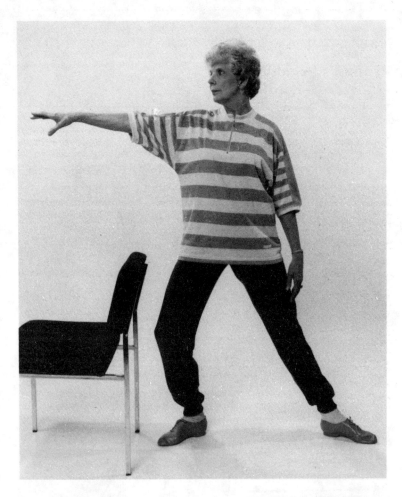

- Very gently bounce three times on the bent leg in this lunge position.
- Straighten both legs.
- Repeat on the other side.
- Carry out this movement four times on both sides.
- To finish, bring your feet together and stand tall.

> Fencing does concentrate a lot on balance. It is important. When you lunge it has to be in a straight line. Another thing is that for older people it is a challenge. It's something that they've probably never done or even tried.
>
> *Tom, 62.*

USEFUL INFORMATION

Ménière's Society
59 Emmanuel Road
London SW12 0HP
01-675 5808
They will provide you with information on how to cope with this distressing disease.

Tranx (UK) Ltd
25A Masons Avenue
Wealdstone
Harrow
Middlesex HA3 5AH
01-247 2065 and 01-247 2827 (24 hours)
Send them a stamped addressed envelope if you want information on their services. If you want help, contact them directly.

Amateur Fencing Association
The De Beauman Centre
83 Perham Road
London W14 9SP
01-385 7442

6
POSTURE

Nothing can make you look older than having a bad posture. Rounded shoulders and a sagging tummy can put years on you. If you sit and stand tall you get more air into your lungs, you give off an air of confidence — and you look slimmer.

BAD POSTURE

As young children we have an almost perfectly straight spine, but as we get older it develops various curves. Most of our bad posture habits are learned in childhood, and our emotions when we are young can affect the way we carry ourselves for the rest of our lives.

If you are embarrassed because you think you are too tall you develop a way of standing with a stoop. If you think your bust is too big, you hunch your shoulders over to cover it. If you feel shy and withdrawn, you curl up.

Bad posture is also caused by wearing shoes with too high a heel, carrying a shoulder bag or a heavy briefcase on one side only, sitting with crossed legs, and sitting on chairs that don't support your back properly.

Bad posture can cause or make worse various health problems. Back pain is the most obvious one, but the wrong posture can also give you migraines, varicose veins, arthritis and rheumatism.

> Since doing t'ai chi I have found a sense of well-being and that's a most valuable thing as you get older because you tend to draw into your self and think about the various aches and pains and stiffnesses and so on. And t'ai chi is good at keeping at bay all of those.
>
> *Donald*, 69.

> If you do the t'ai chi exercises regularly then you become much more aware of your posture, of your trunk, your spine, of your legs, arms, and then you learn to use the trunk and legs and arms and head together. So that it becomes natural. It does give you a great awareness. It's amazing how many people don't realise they've got feet attached to their legs until they do the exercises. And their feet are flexible and legs are flexible rather than just standing on them. And so over a period of a few weeks or months you have a really heightened awareness of your body — probably much more than you've ever had in your life. And so your body becomes softer, your energy flows once you are aware of it and you become like a youngster again.
>
> *Emma*, 67.

GOOD POSTURE

To have a good posture you need to make sure that your centre of gravity is in the right place. Your muscles should be relaxed and you should be able to move freely.

You also need to be able to walk easily. If you have problems with your feet, see a chiropodist. And make sure your shoes are well-fitting.

To balance well you need good co-ordination, and regular exercise will help you to develop this. If you don't normally move around very much you will find that your coordination gets worse.

CHECK YOUR POSTURE

Check yourself to see if your posture could do with some improvement.

- Stand facing a full-length mirror. If one hip and one shoulder is higher than the opposite one, then you are unbalanced.
- Stand with your back to a wall. Touch the wall with your shoulder-blades, calves and heels, and then flatten yourself against it. If you can get your hand between the back of your waist and the wall then you need to improve your posture.

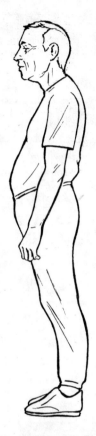

Poor posture

- Face the wall, with your toes touching it. If your head or your stomach are also touching the wall your posture needs some work on it.

CORRECT YOUR POSTURE

To correct your posture you need to be aware of your body, and regular exercise will help you develop that awareness. You need to keep your posture correct at all times — whether you are standing, sitting or lying down. Get your friends to comment of your posture and remind you to keep working on it.

- You should have your head up — and that's the top of your head, not your chin.
- Your weight should be evenly balanced between both feet.
- Your stomach should be pulled in.
- Your shoulders should be relaxed down.
- Your ribs should be held up and open.
- Your knees should be relaxed, not stiff.

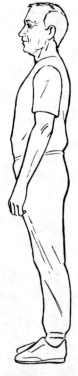

Good posture

I find t'ai chi is of tremendous benefit to older people like me because we generally get into bad postures. We try in the class to soften the body, soften the muscles through breathing exercises, getting the chi energy to flow round the body and this improves the strength.

Arthur, 69.

HELP WITH YOUR POSTURE

Alexander Technique

The Alexander Technique is a method of improving the posture. You will have to go to a specialised teacher who will re-educate your body into a better posture, which will in turn have all sorts of positive side effects — less backache, better breathing, better balance, a more relaxed state of mind.

There is probably at least one Alexander Technique teacher practising near you. If you want to get a list of such teachers, contact the Society of Alexander Technique Teachers.

Osteopathy

Osteopathy can also help to get your spine back into the correct position. It involves a process of very gentle manipulation to put bones and joints back into alignment.

Osteopaths can be found in most parts of the country. If you want the names of ones near you, contact the General Council and Register of Osteopaths.

T'ai chi

T'ai chi was described in the chapter on relaxation, but it is also a very good activity for improving posture and balance. It is actually linked to the ancient Chinese martial arts, but have no fear — you don't have to be a kung fu fighter to learn it.

It is a form of meditation as well as a linked series of movements, and the actions are very graceful and flowing. It exercises every part of the body and teaches a sense of tranquillity and well-being. It is particularly well suited for older people who cannot do more active forms of exercise.

Classes are now quite widely available. Ask at your local library, adult education centre or leisure centre, or contact the British T'ai Chi Ch'uan Association.

Other methods of improving posture

- Yoga has many benefits, but one emphasis is on better posture. This is achieved by relaxing various muscles

and helping to make the joints more supple.
- Massage will help to make you more aware of tense muscles and will relax and invigorate them.
- Chiropractic is similar to osteopathy, in that it involves manipulation of bones and muscles. It can improve posture, restore function to joints and ease pressure on nerves.

WALKING STICK

As you get older you might find that you need a walking stick to help you get around. There is no shame in this and it is sensible to use one if you need it. Your doctor or a physiotherapist should show you the correct way to use it if you have been prescribed one. And don't think you can use any old stick that you've had in the back of the cupboard for years. It might not be the right length for you.

Your stick should reach to the top of your wrist so that you can lean on it without bending over. It should have a rubber tip on the end to stop it slipping, and you should get that replaced regularly.

I tend to have a bad posture on the whole but when it comes to t'ai chi you have to improve it. You can't do the exercises unless you do. So I find it helps with my posture a great deal. I mean this slow breathing, the movements, your posture has to be right or you just can't do it.

Herbert, 70.

I like the stretching exercises because I'm only small and it might make me taller. Who knows. And the bending — I suffer with my back sometimes and it helps with that. I can reach things in the kitchen more easily, get in cupboards without climbing on a stool quite so often, things like that.

Annie, 68.

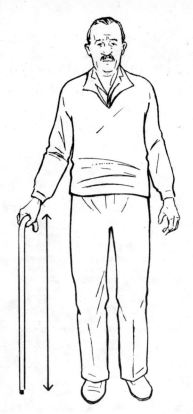

Correct length of a walking stick

EXERCISES TO IMPROVE POSTURE

This selection of exercises is designed to improve your balance, to help avoid internal pressure on your abdominal organs, and to achieve a sense of poise and self-confidence, as well as to lighten the load on your load-bearing joints.

Sitting exercise

You should be sitting tall with your lower back well into the chair and your feet placed comfortably apart.

I had arthritis and I couldn't move easily at all, it was very difficult. But since I started taking regular exercise I feel a lot better in myself, much better, and I'm a lot better for mixing with other people as well.

May, 64

- Curve the middle of your back into the chair, with your head and shoulders slumped slightly forward.
- Slowly straighten your spine until you are sitting tall — your shoulders should be directly over your hips, the

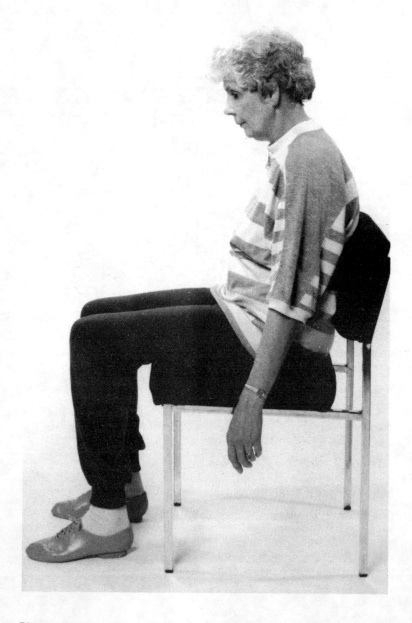

back of your neck stretched, the top of your head lifted towards the ceiling without tipping your chin up.
- Return slowly to the slumped position.

Do this whole exercise four times.

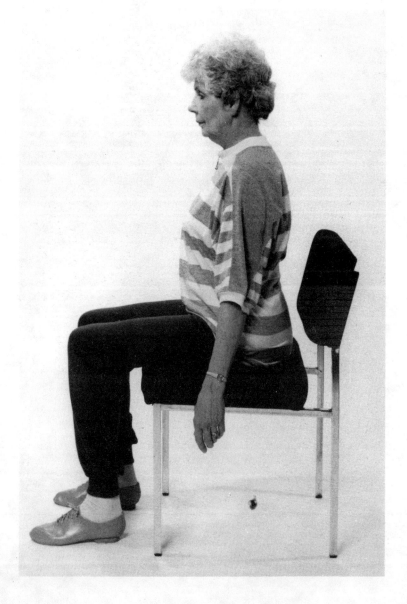

Tummy Muscles
- Sit upright.
- Pull your tummy muscles in.
- Hold for a count of three, then relax.

Repeat this several times, being careful to breathe normally — don't hold your breath.

Head Poise
- Sit up tall in the chair.
- Roll your head forward, then to one side.
- Now roll your head forward again, then to the other side.

Repeat this four times on alternative sides, then return to the tall sitting position and check your posture.

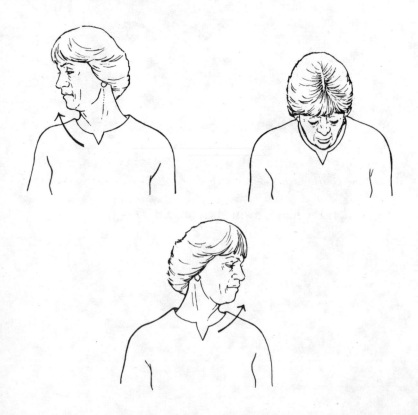

USEFUL INFORMATION

Society of Alexander Technique Teachers
18 Lansdowne Road
London W11
01-272 7222
They will provide you with a list of Alexander Technique teachers practising near you, as well as information on what to expect from the Alexander Technique.

General Council and Register of Osteopaths
21 Suffolk Street
London SW1Y 4HG
01-839 2060
Again, they will tell you of osteopaths practising in your area.

The British T'ai Chi Ch'uan Association
7 Upper Wimpole Street
London W1M 7TD
01-935 8444
They will be able to tell you of the classes they know about in your area.

Alexander Technique, Chris Stevens, Macdonald Optima, £3.95
Osteopathy, Stephen Sandler, Macdonald Optima, £3.95
Chinese Soft Exercise, Paul Crompton, Unwin Hyman, £7.95
T'ai Chi, S P Chia, Unwin Hyman, £6.95

7
BACKS

Back pain affects about 80 per cent of us at some time in our lives, and around 30 million working days are lost each year due to it. But it's never too late to start strengthening your back and introducing some suppleness into it — you shouldn't think that having a bad back is an inevitable consequence of growing older.

THE SPINE

There are 110 joints in the spine, linked by a covering membrane. The spine itself consists of 33 bones stacked on top of one another, with gristly discs between them to act as shock absorbers. These individual bones — the vertebrae — and discs form a flexible column from the neck to the small of the back.

Furthermore, the spinal cord — a thick bundle of nerves — runs inside this spinal column, with nerves radiating off to various parts of the body. Small wonder then that the back can be so easily damaged and that the damage can sometimes have such far-reaching effects on other parts of the body.

BACK PAIN

Back pain can be caused by many different things — illness, injury, even emotional stress.

- The discs between the vertebrae can be damaged, or slip out of position.
- Sciatica can be caused by pressure on the roots of the nerves in the spine.
- The bones can move out of alignment.

- Joints can be come inflamed.
- The muscles around the spine can go into spasm and lock up because of a sprain or bad posture.

Even corns on your feet can cause back problems, by forcing you to stand incorrectly and so putting strain on your back.

So you should always get back pain checked by your doctor — it could be a symptom of something serious such as kidney disease or gallstones.

However, most bad backs are caused because we don't treat them with the respect and care they deserve. If we did, then a lot of that pain could be avoided.

HELPING YOUR BACK

Learn to improve your posture — read Chapter 6 on posture.

- Make sure that work-surfaces, desk, ironing boards, etc., are at the correct height for you so you are not continually bending over.

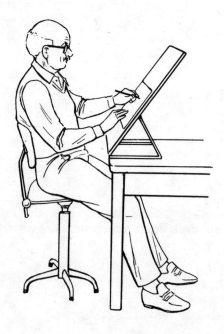

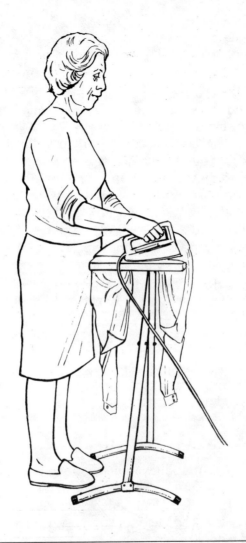

When you're older you tend not to do quite as much exercise. But you move every part of your body in swimming and use every muscle. It loosens you up all over, particularly your back. It's good for breathing as well.

Harriet, 64.

I've always loved the water. It's nice and easy — all your limbs are free.

Lucy, 70.

- Make sure that your chair gives your back the right support.
- Your bed shouldn't be too soft. If it is and you can't buy a new mattress, get a board put under the old one to make it firmer.
- Make sure your shoes fit properly and that your feet don't hurt. Painful feet can affect your posture.
- Learn the correct way to lift and carry things. For example, don't put all your shopping in one bag — divide it between two and carry one in each hand. If you use a shopping bag on wheels push it in front of you — don't drag it along.
- Always bend at the knees and keep your back straight when picking something up. Lift a heavy bag by crouching over it, picking it up with both hands and holding it close to your chest, and then straighten the knees as you stand up. Reverse all this to put it down again.
- Keep your weight down so your spine has less to support.
- Don't drag heavy furniture around — push against it with your back instead. And get help to move things if you need it.

EXERCISE AND YOUR BACK

To support your spine you need strong back and stomach muscles, as well as strong legs to take the strain when you lift something. Gentle regular exercise will strengthen these muscles, while learning to relax will help if your bad back is due to tension.

Swimming, keep-fit classes and yoga can all be beneficial. In fact, swimming is probably the best all-round exercise you can do; it builds your strength, stamina and suppleness, and because the water supports your body you are unlikely to strain any muscles. It's also widely available — most towns have a swimming pool — and quite cheap.

HELP FOR YOUR BACK

There are many people you can now turn to for help if you have a bad back — or if you want to avoid getting a bad back.

Physiotherapy can help with back problems, either through the NHS or privately. If you want to see a physiotherapist, contact your GP or write to the Chartered Society of Physiotherapists.

We have already mentioned the Alexander Technique in previous chapters. Teachers of this method believe that a lot of backache is caused by poor posture resulting from physical or emotional stress. Their treatment aims to reduce problems in the back by restoring correct posture.

Similarly an osteopath or a chiropractitioner may be able to solve your back problem by manipulation.

And there are a number of specialist shops that sell furniture, beds, pillows, etc., specifically designed to ease or remove back problems.

The Back Pain Association

As an indication of how common back pain is, there is now an association aimed at linking together sufferers of back problems, running self-help groups, giving advice and distributing information.

If you want to find about more about the Back Pain Association, contact them directly.

EXERCISES FOR YOUR BACK

Strengthen your back
- Stand up straight with your arms by your sides.
- Bend your arms and bring your hands together in front of your chest.

Well I think you can move better when you've been in the water, and you feel better in the water. It does you good ... it's better than sitting at home watching television isn't it.
Aileen, 57.

- Stretch your hands and arms forward as if you're doing the breaststroke.

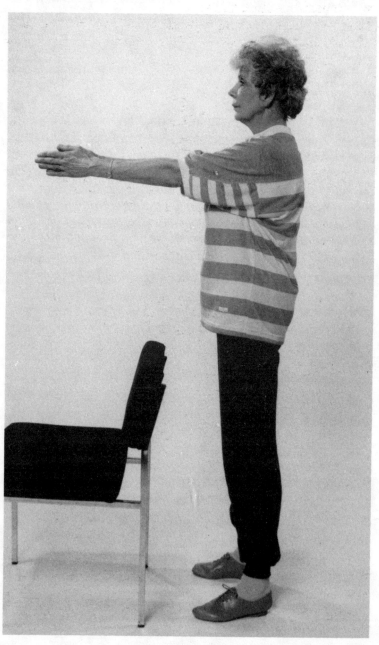

- Open your arms out to the sides at shoulder height.
- Gently drop your arms back down to your sides.
- Repeat this three times.

Ease your back by doing a gentle knee bend, holding on to a chair-back if necessary. Then repeat the movement three more times.

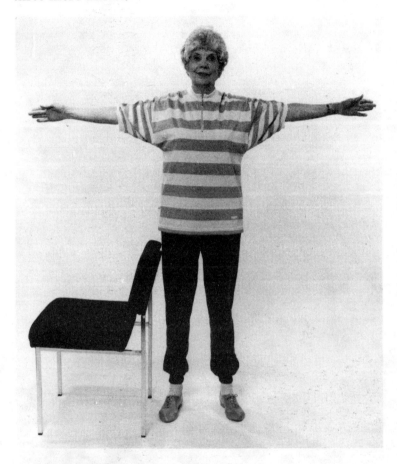

Exercise for the lower back

Stand up straight with both hands on the back of a chair. You should keep your hands on the chair during this exercise, although you can feel the position of the back by putting a hand over the small of the back before starting the movements.

- Slide the left leg behind you, with the toes bent.
- Keep the weight on your forward leg and bend it slightly.

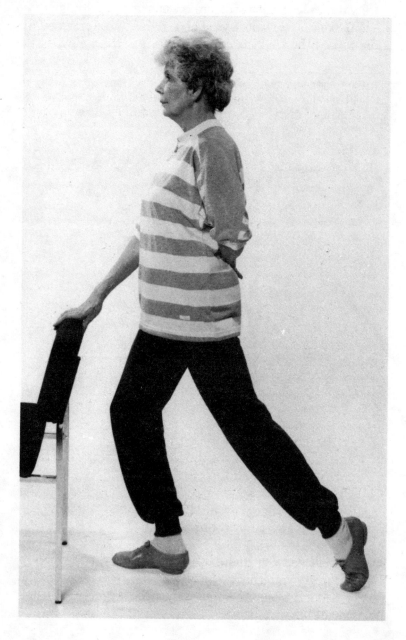

- Brace your shoulders and hold this bent-leg position for a count of three.
- Repeat the movement with the other leg.
- Do the movement two more times with each leg.
- Release any tension with eight walks on the spot.

Then repeat the whole exercise, starting with the left leg.

When I started swimming I was very frightened to go into the deep end but my friends persuaded me. They go one on each side of me you see. I'm better than the Queen in the water you know.

Jeannie, 63.

I've had two frozen shoulders and a trapped nerve, and I wear a steel corset. I have a bad back and swimming's done me good.

Helen, 66.

The infirmary told me the best exercise was swimming and I've found it a big benefit. You seem to use your arms more and it keeps you in trim. I've had a lot of pleasure from swimming, it doesn't hurt any more and I don't go for treatment any more.

Ethel, 72.

Exercise for the upper back

Stand tall with your hands on a chair-back, feet comfortably apart, legs straight.

- Lift one hand and place it lightly on the same shoulder, with your elbow relaxed.
- Lift the elbow a little way to the front.
- Take the elbow round to the side, keeping the shoulder down and relaxed all the time.
- Take the elbow as far back as you can, pulling the elbow down towards the back and slightly turning the trunk in the same direction.
- Do this three times.
- Then place both hands on the chair and gently bend your knees to remove any tension.

Repeat the exercise with the other arm, again relaxing at the end with a knee bend.

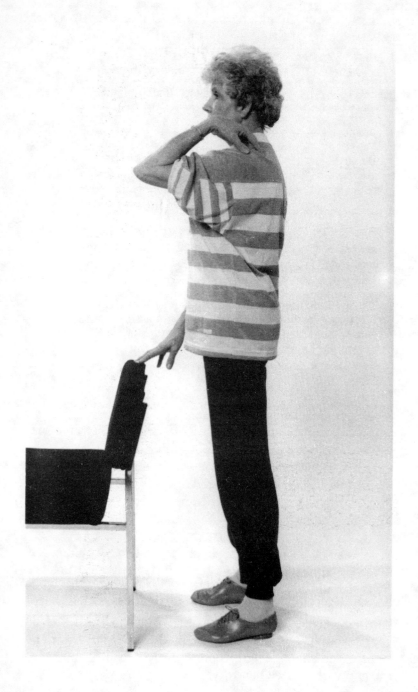

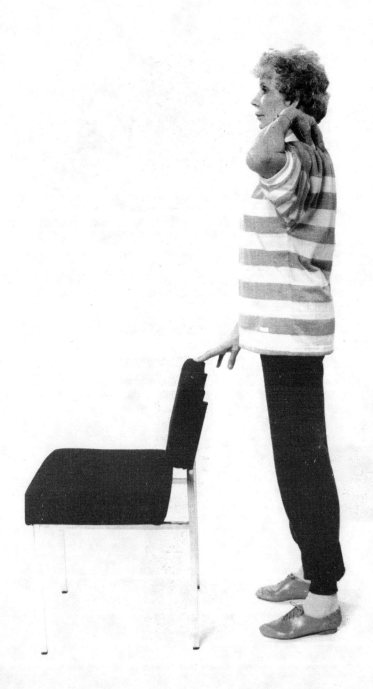

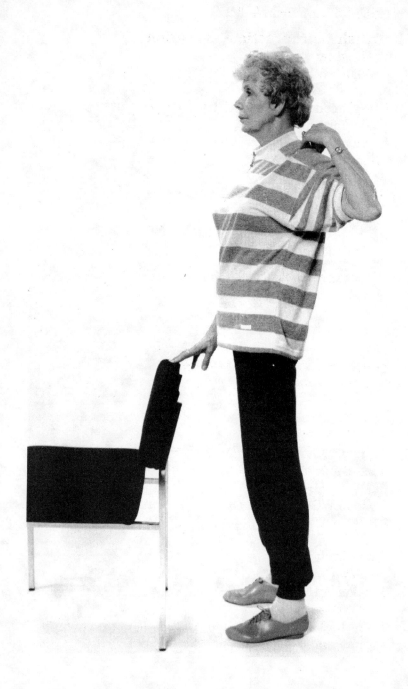

USEFUL INFORMATION

British Chiropractic Association
10 Greycoat Place
London SW1P 1SB

Chartered Society of Physiotherapists
14 Bedford Row
London WC1R 4ED
01-242 1941

Society of Alexander Teachers
18 Lansdowne Road
London W11
01-272 7222

General Council and Register of Osteopaths
21 Suffolk Street
London SW1Y 4HG
01-839 2060

National Back Pain Association
31–3 Park Road
Teddington
Middlesex TW11 0AB
01-977 5474/5

The Back Store
324 King Street
London W6
01-741 5022

The Back Shop
24 New Cavendish Street
London W1M 7LH
01-934 9120
Both these shops stock a wide range of products to prevent and relieve back problems.

Chiropractic, Susan Moore, Macdonald Optima, £3.95
Alexander Technique, Chris Stevens, Macdonald Optima, £3.95
Osteopathy, Stephen Sandler, Macdonald Optima, £3.95
The Back: Relief from Pain, Dr Alan Stoddard, Macdonald Optima/Positive Health Guides, £5.99

8
HANDS, ARMS AND SHOULDERS

One of the biggest problems we can have when we are older is that our hands start to stiffen up with arthritis or rheumatism, and without the use of our hands we lose a lot of our independence. It is thought that about one person in seven suffers from arthritis — rheumatoid arthritis, osteoarthritis and gout — at some point during their lives and women are twice as likely to get it as men.

But doing simple exercises with your hands every day should help to keep them supple.

HELPFUL TIPS

If you suffer from arthritis in your hands, here are some simple tips to make life a bit easier around the house.

- Use a paper clip through the tab of a zip to help you get a better grip on it to pull the zip up and down.
- Sew some cloth loops on to the tops of your socks to make them easier to pull up.
- Don't use heavy saucepans and dishes in the kitchen — buy some lighter ones.
- Use felt-tip pens instead of ballpoints — they need less pressure to make them write.
- Don't struggle to hold up your newspaper while you are reading it — lay it flat on the table in front of you.
- Keep your hands warm — always wear gloves in the winter.

There are a lot of very useful gadgets available now to help in everyday life. There are dustpans and brushes with long handles so you don't have to bend over, large-grip knives, forks, spoons and kitchen implements, and aids to help you get dressed such as shoe horns, hooks to pull up zips and so on.

For the kitchen there are non-slip bowls and spiked chopping boards which hold the food steady while you are preparing it. There is also a very useful thing called a gripper or arm extender, which you can use to pick things up from the floor or to reach from high shelves.

A lot of these gadgets are on sale in good hardware stores. In some areas the Social Services Department will supply them for you. Even if you can't get them free, the Social Services will tell you where you can buy them, so contact them for the address of your local supplier.

CAN I PREVENT ARTHRITIS?

Research has shown that taking evening primrose oil can considerably help relieve the symptoms for some sufferers of rheumatoid arthritis. You could try taking three 500-mg tablets twice a day. It is available from chemists and health-food stores.

Calcium has also been found to be of benefit. You may find that taking six to nine bonemeal tablets daily helps you, or you could try Dolomite tablets which combine calcium with magnesium. These too are available from chemists and health-food stores.

If you want more information about arthritis and tips to help live with it write to Arthritis Care.

SIMPLE EXERCISES

These exercises are well worth doing every day to keep your hands supple. Don't forget that even if you are stuck in a chair or in bed every day, you can still work on your hands.

- Tightly clench your fist. Then unclench it and stretch your fingers apart as wide as you can. Repeat ten times on each hand.

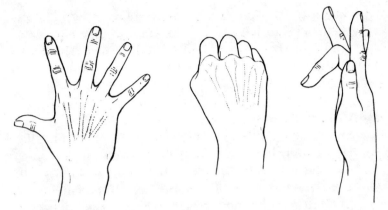

- Bend one finger at a time into the palm of your hand, keeping the other fingers straight.
- Shake your hands from the wrists, up and down and round and round, until they feel limp and relaxed.
- Squeeze a soft rubber ball in the palm of your hand to exercise the muscles in your hand, wrist and forearm.

EXTEND

EXTEND stands for Exercise Training for the Elderly and Disabled, and they organise a wide range of classes throughout the country to help elderly and disabled people keep fit and retain as much mobility as possible.

If you do not know of any classes near you, contact EXTEND and they will let you know of what's available.

The classes will certainly keep you on the move and, perhaps just as importantly, allow you to meet other people who are keen on keeping fit and active.

MASSAGE AND TOUCH

Touching is something many of us have got out of the habit of doing, but it can express as many emotions as words. If you live on your own or in an old people's home, perhaps because your husband or wife has died, it can be very easy to get through the day with no real contact with other people.

Sometimes, if your living circumstances permit, it is very beneficial to have a pet, particularly a cat or a dog that you can stroke and cuddle. Getting together with a friend and giving each other a hand massage can be even more comforting and can relieve a lot of stress.

Hand massage

Massage is an excellent way of keeping your hands supple. Here is a simple hand massage you could try on yourself or on someone else, although remember not to try it if the joints of the hand are swollen, painful or inflamed.

- Pinch firmly all round the outer edge of the hand.
- Pinch gently in the fleshy area between the thumb and forefinger.
- Knead into the palm of the hand with your fist.
- Using your thumb and index finger, make small circling movements round each joint, beginning at the base of each finger and working up. When you get to the tip of each finger, pull it gently.
- Stroke firmly from the wrists down to the knuckles between each pair of tendons on the back of the hand.
- Use almond oil when you massage your hands. It is very pleasant and is cheap and easily available at the chemist.

Hand massage is particularly soothing for someone who is ill in bed. Perhaps when you are visiting a friend in hospital and they don't feel much like talking — it's nice to give them a gentle hand massage then.

EXERCISES FOR HANDS, ARMS AND SHOULDERS

Mobilise and strengthen the hands

Sit in a chair with your arms in their natural position, relaxed on your thighs.

I didn't think the exercises would work, but now that I've done them and got my wrists working properly, I'd recommend them to anybody.

Emily, 63.

- Lift your lower arms slightly.
- Hold up the palms of your hands so your fingers are pointing towards the ceiling.
- Then clench and unclench your hands, spreading your fingers wide apart as you unclench them.

Do this eight times.

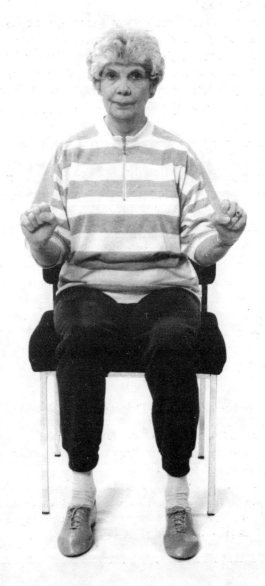

> I couldn't put my wrists together, I couldn't do that at all, no way, now I can move them. It's been a great help. I feel much more mobile.
>
> *May, 72.*

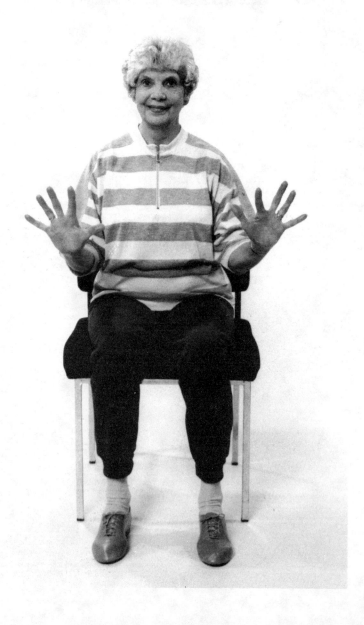

Wrists

Sit in a chair as before.

- Raise the palms of your hands, with the fingers together. Then drop the hands and raise them again, four times, working from the wrists.

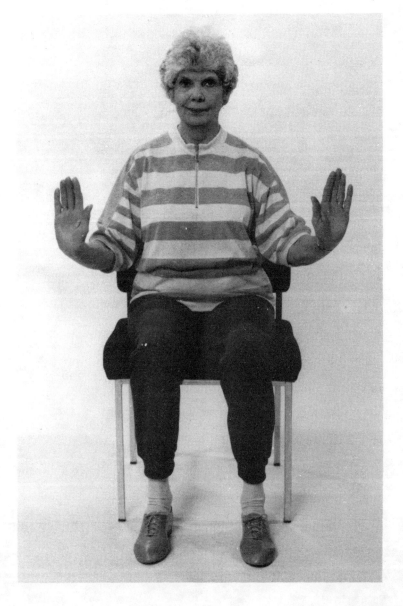

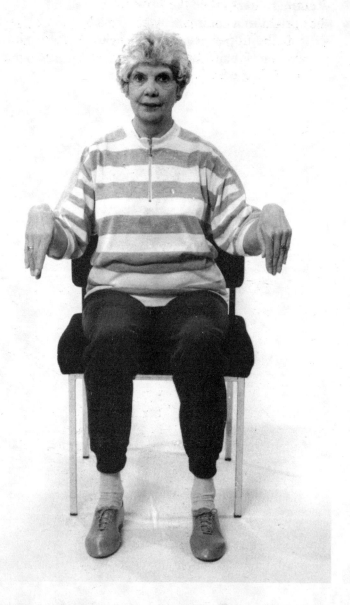

- With the palms raised as before, circle the hands from the wrists, twice one way then twice the other way.
- Relax and shake your hands, arms gently by your sides.

Arms (Helps to tone the upper arms.)

Sit upright in a chair with your arms by your sides.

- Lift the upper arms to just below shoulder level. The elbows should be bent, the hands hanging down towards the floor.

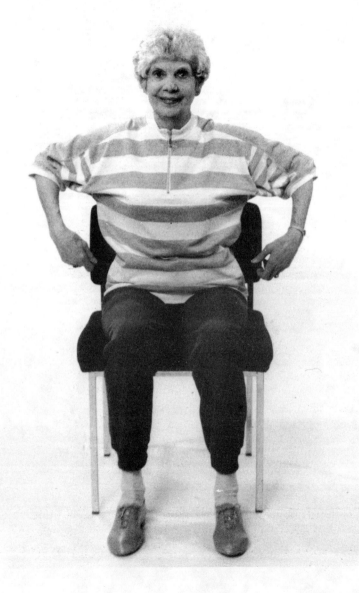

- Stretch both arms out to the sides at shoulder level.
- Reverse the movement, bending the elbows, allowing the hands to drop, then sliding the arms down to either side of the body.

Do this movement four times.

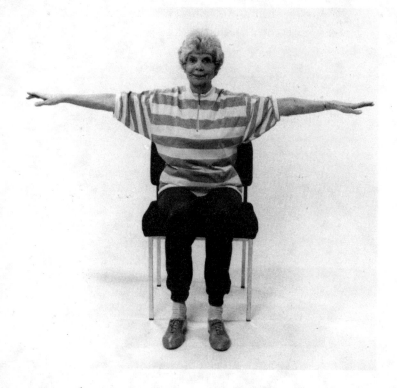

My left arm was bad with arthritis and I couldn't lift it up. So I started just lifting it a little bit and a little bit ... and finally after a fortnight I got so that I could lift my arm straight up. I gave my husband the shock of his life, 'cos I was saving it as a surprise.

Dot, 70.

I broke my arm a few years ago and it wasn't set properly. But since I've been doing the exercises I can do all my own gardening, push the lawnmower.

Irene, 60.

Shoulders

Again, sit up tall in a chair with your arms down by your sides.

- Pull one shoulder up towards the ear, keeping the head still and trying not to move any other part of your body.
- Slowly relax the shoulder down to its normal position.
- Repeat with the other shoulder.

Do the whole exercise four times.

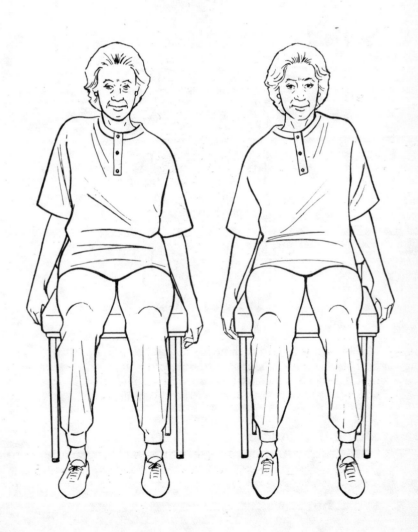

- Now raise both shoulders to your ears, then lower them slowly to the starting position. Do this twice.

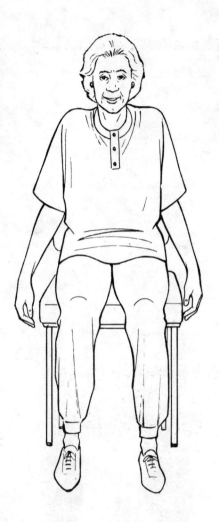

Arms and Shoulders
Sit up straight in a chair with a headscarf or square in your hands.
- Stretch the scarf between your hands so that your arms are opened out.

- Lift your arms over your head with the scarf still under tension.

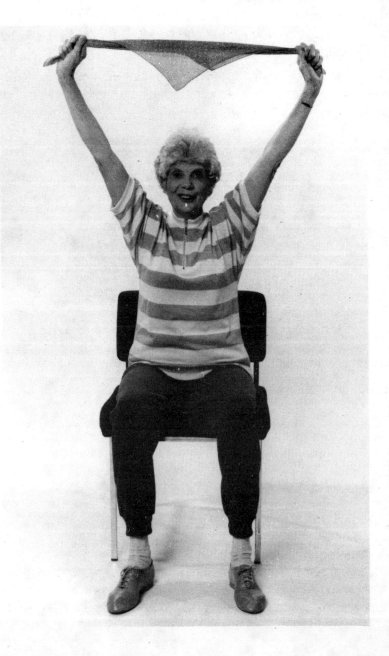

- Bend your elbows and lower the scarf down behind your head — if this proves too tough, bring it down in front of your face.
- Straighten your arms again, then lower them down in front of you, keeping the scarf under tension all the time.

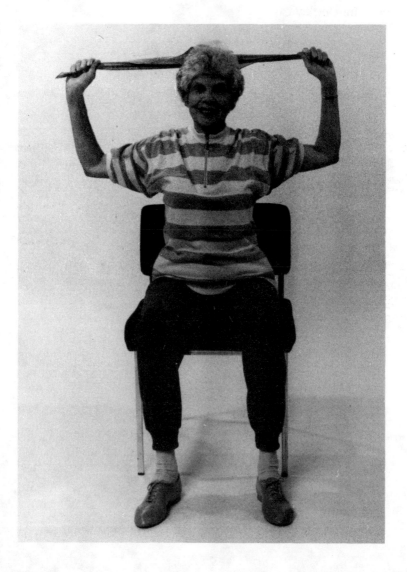

USEFUL INFORMATION

Arthritis Care
6 Grosvenor Crescent
London SW1X 7ER
01-235 0902

EXTEND
3 The Boulevard
Sheringham
Norfolk
NR26 8LJ
0263 822479

League of Health and Beauty
18 Charing Cross Road
London WC2 0HR
01-240 8456

Overcoming Arthritis, Dr Frank Dudley Hart, Macdonald
Optima/Positive Health Guides, £4.99
Answers to Arthritis, Tony van den Bergh, Macdonald
Optima, £3.95
Why Endure Rheumatism and Arthritis? Clifford Quick,
Unwin Hyman, £2.95

9
HIPS

As we get older our hips can give us a lot of trouble. We fall over and break them, we get arthritis in them — and some of us even end up with new plastic and metal ones.

TROUBLESOME HIPS

The main function of the hip joint is to bear the weight of our body when we are in an upright position, and in every movement where we are transferring our weight from one leg to the other.

As we grow older the hip joints, in common with all our other joints, suffer from wear and tear, osteoarthritis or other problems. Joints that have been injured at some time during our life are particularly likely to cause trouble in old age, especially if they have to support a lot of weight. If the hips suffer in this way it can lead to severe pain and loss of mobility.

PROTECT YOUR HIPS

We can protect our hip joints by keeping our weight down to as near our ideal as possible — carrying too much weight around puts unnecessary strain on the hips. We should also develop an awareness of how we actually treat our joints and how we can make life easier for them — and for us.

For example, if you have to stand for a long time, perhaps while waiting for a bus or in a queue at the super-market, do you put all your weight on one leg? If you do, you are throwing your hips out of line and putting too much strain on to just one of them. Be aware of your stance and make sure you are standing with your weight evenly distributed on both legs.

If you can't do that for some reason, then walk up and down occasionally, or transfer your weight from one foot to the other to relieve the tension and keep the circulation going. Alternatively, you could flex your calf muscles while standing still, first one calf then the other — this will help the blood circulation and reduce the feeling of tiredness. Having a good posture and deep breathing will help here.

If you get very tired when you stand, rest on your bed when you can, to take the weight off your hips, knees and feet. Your bed should be firm to support your spine properly. And when you sit, don't cross your legs — this is bad for the hips and can interfere with the blood supply in the legs, often leading to varicose veins.

GET A GOOD CHAIR

If you have problems with your hips, you may well spend a lot of time sitting in a chair. It is therefore very important that the chair you are in is supporting you properly.

The seat needs to be deep enough to support the whole of your upper leg from knee to hip. It should be comfortable but not sagging. The height of the seat should allow you to place your feet flat on the floor with your thighs supported on the seat.

The back of the chair should be tall enough to accommodate the shape of your spine and support the back of your head. The chair should be wide enough for comfort and have arms which you can easily rest your lower arms on.

> I had a hip replacement and I've hurt my ankle, so when I walk any distance or carry anything the pain is very bad. But when I dance, you see someone is holding me when I dance and it just takes the weight off I suppose. And I enjoy it so much that the pain becomes less.
>
> *Selina*, 79.

HOW TO USE A CHAIR

It can be very difficult to get in and out of a chair that is too deep or low. Here is how you should do it.

Walk up to the chair and turn so your back is towards it. Feel the chair with the back of your lower leg. Leaning forward slightly let yourself down gently into the seat. As your knees bend, reach for the arms with your hands. You may need to shuffle backwards on your bottom to get to the back of the seat.

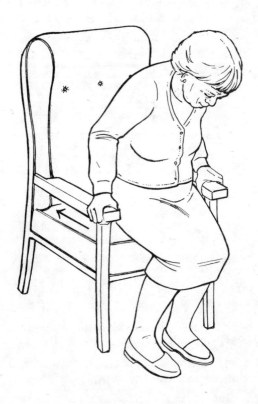

It keeps you fit and it keeps you young. And when you go round a dance floor and you arc trying to do what you did 40 years ago and you've got this bevy of beauties round you it's lovely!

Gordon, 78.

When you're in the chair, sit tall and try not to slump. Don't cross your legs — it's not good for the hip joints and it puts pressure on the veins in your legs.

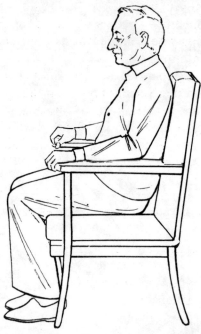

And when you come to get up again, get up slowly and steadily. Place one foot slightly in front of the other and very slightly bend forward. With your hands on the chair arms, gently take your weight on to your feet. Straighten your knees and make sure you are balanced.

OSTEOPOROSIS

The reason why many older women suffer from a broken hip after what may seem at the time like a minor tumble is that they suffer from a condition called osteoporosis. As we get older our bones start to lose calcium and become more brittle, making them more likely to break. This process happens a lot faster after the menopause.

Regular exercise can actually replace the calcium and strengthen the bones. Researchers have found that women aged 50 to 62 who did aerobics three times a week for a year actually increased the calcium level in their bones by 4 per cent while those of a similar age who did not exercise at all lost 1 per cent of their bone calcium.

So it really is worthwhile taking up regular exercise as early in your life as you can to ward off the risk of breaking your hips when older. But as the research shows, it is never too late to start.

It is also a good idea to make sure that you are eating a calcium-rich diet (or perhaps even taking calcium supplements). Foods with a high calcium content are milk, cheese, yogurt and all other dairy products, eggs, sardines (including the bones), wholemeal bread, broccoli, spring cabbage, watercress, oranges, peanuts, brazil nuts and baked beans.

In order to absorb the calcium efficiently, we also need enough vitamin D. We get this from two main sources — sunlight, or eggs, liver, seafish and some cereals to which extra vitamin D has been added. However, if you decide to take a vitamin D supplement don't exceed more than 10 mg a day as too much can harm your health. Consult your doctor about this.

AFTER A HIP OPERATION

If you do have the misfortune to break a bone or have a hip replacement operation, it is important to exercise regularly as soon as possible afterwards.

The physiotherapist in the hospital will help you with exercises before you leave, and will recommend exercises you can continue with at home. And the sooner you start on these exercises, the sooner you'll get back to normal, although you ought to take your doctor's advice on when you can begin.

DANCING

Going to an exercise class will help keep your hip joints mobile, but such classes are only one way of taking exercise.

Sometimes it's nice to make it more of a social occasion, and that's where ballroom, sequence or oldtime dancing can be useful; tea dances, for example, are held all over the country every day of the week. The music and the company make you forget that you are actually exercising your hips.

STRENGTHEN YOUR HIPS AND BACK

Here is a good hip exercise which will also help to strengthen your back.

Lie on one side with your head resting on a pillow. One arm should be comfortably underneath you and the other either on the bed in front of you or holding the side of the bed to prevent you rolling over.

- Bend the top leg without lifting it.
- Stretch the leg forward over the edge of the bed as far as you can.
- Keeping the leg straight, move it back past the stationary leg as far as you can. You will find that the leg will only go a very little way back beyond the other leg because that is all the movement in that direction that the hip can manage. If you push it back a little bit further you will feel your lower back working.
- Providing that it is comfortable, repeat the movement three or four times before you roll over to do the same with the other leg.

> Dancing helps me immensely. I'm very, very lame, I have to walk with a stick and I need a new hip replacement, but once I'm dancing and the music starts I'm just as fit as a fiddle really.
>
> *Frank*, 79.

EXERCISES FOR YOUR HIPS

Lie on your back with your head supported by a pillow and with both knees bent, feet on the bed. Keep your spine against the bed and don't hollow your back.

- Bring one knee towards your chest.
- Straighten the leg overhead.
- Bend the leg.
- Put it down beside the other leg.
- Repeat several times with each leg.

Now try the same exercise from a lying position where your legs are straight out on the bed. Be careful not to hollow your back and make sure you keep your tummy muscles very gently pulled in.

Now try this exercise lying on your back with your arms out to the sides to stop you rolling over, and your legs straight.

- Bend one knee on to your chest.
- Keeping the knee bent, take the leg out to the side,
- Bring the knee back to the chest.
- Keeping the knee bent, take it across the body.
- Bring the knee back to the chest.
- Replace the leg on the bed.
- Repeat with the other leg.

I've always enjoyed dancing and since I found I had a blocked artery I try and come more because the doctor said it would help. I used to do keep-fit exercises but I think it is more enjoyable to dance. And I think it has helped to improve my leg a lot; it doesn't ache as much now as it did. The doctor said it could get better without having an operation.

Maud, 74.

I'm very bad with my feet with arthritis, and dancing has worked wonders for me. I actually have no trace of it at all now, y'know. Dance the night away as you might say. Dancing has done me good, yes.

Wilf, 80.

HIPS AND LEG EXERCISES

Turning the leg

Stand to one side of a chair and check your upright position — stand tall with your feet slightly apart and straight towards the front.

Hold the chair with the hand nearest it and turn the left foot, leg and hip out as far as comfortable.
- Turn it back towards the front.
- Repeat with the right leg and foot.
- Do this eight times with alternate legs.

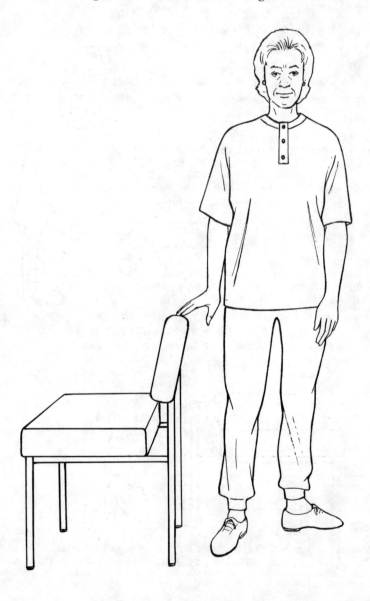

Bending the leg

Take up the same position again to the side of the chair.

- Now bend the left knee and lift the left leg up and across the right leg.

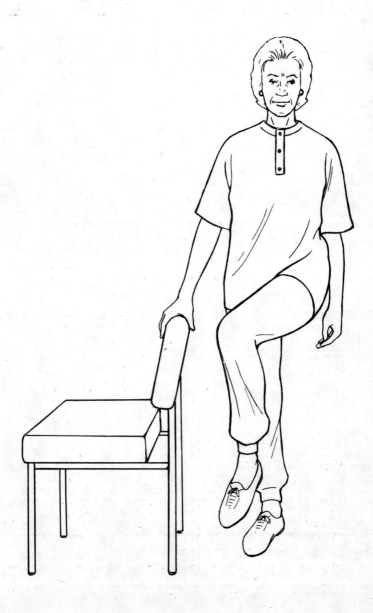

- Take the left leg back then stretch it out to the left side, with the toe on the floor.

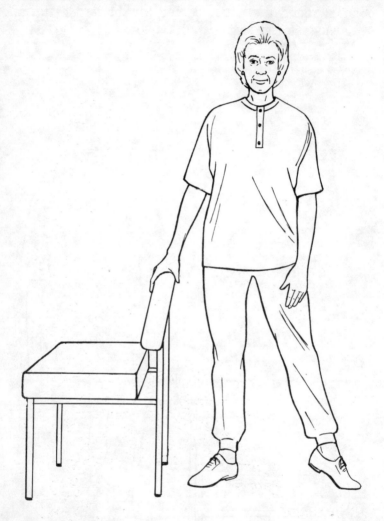

- Repeat the lift across.
- Replace the foot back on the floor with the weight on both feet.
- Repeat with the other leg.
- Do the whole sequence four times using alternate legs, and being careful not to kick the chair with the leg next to it.

Swinging the leg
Again take up the same standing position to the side of the chair.

* Swing the left leg forward and back from the hip —

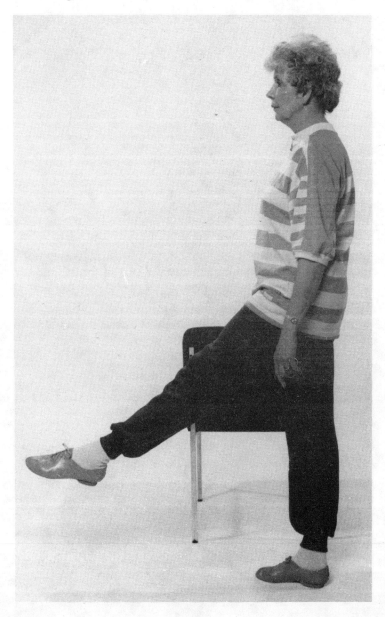

you should have a straight leg, a steady trunk and the supporting leg should be straight. Don't swing too high.

- Do three complete swings and then rest.
- Do three complete swings with the other leg.

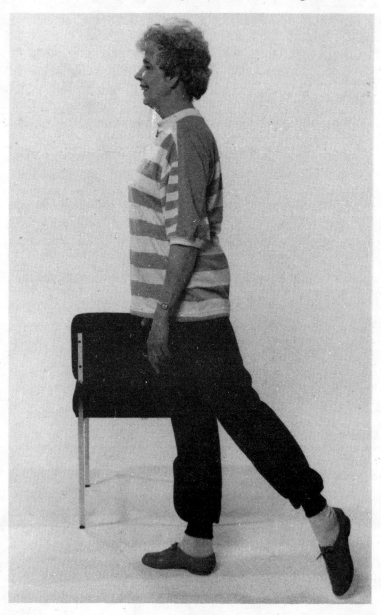

Again, make sure you are far enough away from the chair not to kick it.

STRETCHING AND WAIST EXERCISES

Back curling
Sit up tall in a chair, with your lower back well into the chair and your feet placed flat on the floor, comfortably apart.

- Curve the middle of your back into the base of the chair, with your head and shoulders slumped slightly forwards.
- Slowly straighten your spine until you are sitting tall again, your shoulders directly over your hips, the back of your neck stretched, and the top of your head stretched up to the ceiling without your chin being tipped up.
- Slowly return to the slumped position.
- Do this two times.

You will remember that this is also one of the exercises for good posture from Chapter Six.

I notice a difference when I'm going to exercise classes. I think it helps to keep you more supple, even about your ordinary housework, your bending and stretching – it's so much easier.

Gladys, 63.

Side bending (see page 120)
- Remaining in the tall position gently bend to the right from the waist — the ear should be over the shoulder and the shoulder over the hip.
- Gently straighten up, then repeat on the left side.
- Do this movement four times on alternate sides, sitting up tall in between.

Here is a variation on this movement if you want a greater
stretch.
* Repeat the side bend as before.

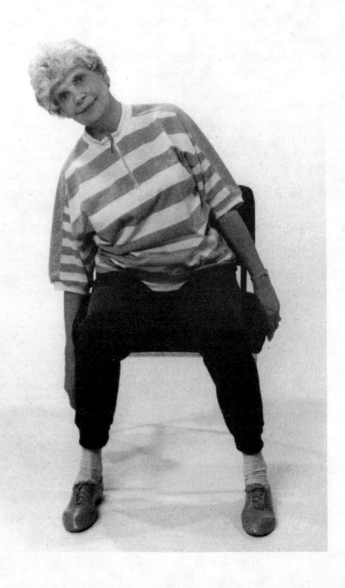

- As one arm reaches towards the floor on the bending side, the other arm bends with the elbow towards the ceiling and with the hand sliding into the armpit.
- Again, repeat this movement four times on alternate sides, but only if the stretch isn't too strong.

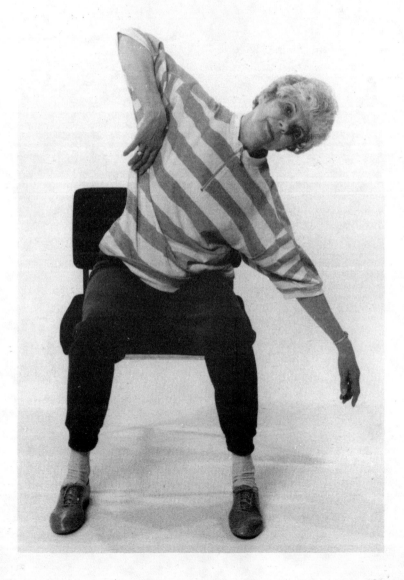

Forward bend

Again, start in the tall sitting position, with the top of the head up towards the ceiling.

- Bend forward from the hips, with a straight flat back. The arms should be behind you, towards the chair back, with the shoulder-blades flattened.
- Return to the tall upright position.
- Relax the spine, curling it into the base of the chair.
- Sit up straight and tall again.

Do this movement twice in all.

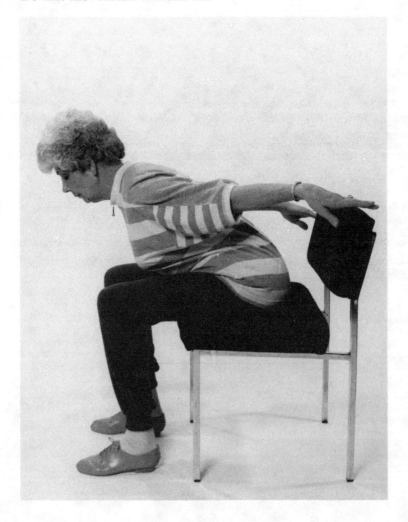

USEFUL INFORMATION

National Osteoporosis Society
Barton Meade House
PO Box 10
Radstock
Bath BA3 3YB

Provide information on diet, calcium-rich foods, Hormone
Replacement Therapy, exercise.

10
FEET AND LEGS

Your feet contain a quarter of the body's bones, and each foot has 19 muscles and 115 ligaments. Furthermore, by the time we reach 70 most of us will have walked about 75,000 miles — roughly three times round the world.

So you can understand why your feet and legs need a bit of attention from time to time.

EXERCISE YOUR FEET AND LEGS

Walking is one of the best forms of exercise for your feet and legs. And what's more, it is also good for all the other parts of you — it makes your heart, lungs and circulation work more efficiently, can help you lose weight, tones up your whole body, prevents varicose veins and reduces swollen legs and ankles.

If you want to go on organised walks you could contact the Ramblers' Association. Or maybe you'd prefer to go cycling or dancing — they're both good for your feet and legs, too.

LOOK AFTER YOUR FEET

It is important to look after your feet. Wash them every day and dry them thoroughly, including between the toes. Keep the nails short — cut them straight across to avoid ingrowing toenails.

Aching feet can be caused by wearing badly-fitting shoes, being overweight, or by having a bad posture. Go barefooted whenever you can. Try to buy leather shoes which allow the feet to breathe, and make sure your shoes are comfortable and suitable for your purposes. Keep your feet warm.

FOOT MASSAGE

Foot massage is very soothing and relaxing. You can do it yourself or ask someone else to do it for you. It improves the circulation in the foot and relaxes the muscles.

Almond oil from the chemist is a good oil to use for massage, or you could try one of the special foot creams — peppermint is particularly soothing. Here's how to do a foot massage.

- Massage the instep and the heel of the foot.
- Squeeze each toe firmly between the thumb and fore-finger.
- Press firmly between the bones at the base of the foot.
- Clasp the toes with your hand and bend them towards you. Release and repeat.
- Gently pull each of the toes away from its neighbour.
- Using your thumb and index finger, make small circling movements around each toe joint, beginning at the base and working upwards.
- When you reach the tip of the toe, pull it gently and squeeze the flesh around the nail and the nail pad.

WHERE TO GET HELP

If you are having trouble with your feet ask your doctor to refer you to a chiropodist (free to pensioners on the NHS). Or you can go privately, but you'll have to pay.

Your local telephone directory and Citizens Advice Bureau will have names and addresses of chiropodists near you, or you can contact the Society of Chiropodists — they have information on all foot problems, and lists of chiropodists.

I like the soothing rhythm of the music that sends you round. But another thing I like is that you've got to think a little. And it's really very good, you know, to exercise your mind. That's what I really like about it. And they're nice gentle easy steps which are easy on your feet as well. It's lovely. I'd recommend it to anybody, men especially.

Alice, 68.

LEG PROBLEMS

Varicose veins

Varicose veins are a problem of poor circulation. If you suffer from them you should always try to put your legs up — on a stool or another chair — whenever you sit down. And don't cross them — this puts pressure on the veins and can increase the problem.

Gentle massage of the legs helps, although you shouldn't put too much pressure on them. And gently applying a little lemon juice is also said to be a good remedy.

You can get support stockings and tights very easily now, either on the NHS or in the shops. There are some new lightweight ones available that are very attractive, so you don't have to look frumpy.

Cramp

Cramp can be a very painful problem, particularly if it strikes at night.

More vitamin E can help reduce cramps, as can anything that helps to improve the blood circulation — exercise and massage, for example. A relaxation technique may also help.

Once you've got cramp, the best way to relieve it is to stretch the cramped muscle gently. For instance if the back of your calf is cramped, you can ease it out by straightening your leg and pointing your toes towards your face.

PROBLEMS WITH FEET

Three of the most common problems with feet are bunions, chilblains and corns.

Bunions

A bunion is the swollen joint of the big toe and it can be very painful. Soaking the feet daily in one tablespoon of Epsom salts dissolved in warm water can ease it, as can gently massaging the joint, although don't do that if it is inflamed and hot.

Try to keep the joint from stiffening up by exercising it gently while you are having a bath, as the warmth will help to ease it.

Chilblains

Chilblains are caused by bad circulation and can be eased by taking more exercise. Massaging the feet can increase the circulation, and you could try rubbing calendula cream (made from marigolds) gently on to the chilblains. Taking extra vitamin E (which is good for skin problems) and vitamin C may help too.

Corns

Corns are often a big problem for older people and can make getting around very difficult. Try to prevent them from developing in the first place by rubbing areas of hard skin with a pumice stone regularly and softening them with vitamin E cream.

More importantly, make sure your shoes fit properly and see a chiropodist if necessary.

EXERCISES FOR THE FEET AND LEGS

Leg lifts

This exercise is particularly good for the legs and abdomen. You should be sat up straight in a chair, with a headscarf or square to hand.

> Dancing's strengthened my legs and made the muscles more supple. I can crouch down now and I haven't been able to do that for years.
>
> *Jim, 75.*
>
> Well, because of an earlier injury, my leg was rather weak and I got arthritis which stiffened up the knee. But since I've been to the dancing it has eased it. And I've never been able to let myself go before, so I've never learned how to dance. But here I feel we're all one and we can all make mistakes together and not feel silly about it.
>
> *Ellen, 71.*

- Take the scarf in the right hand.
- Lift the right leg and swing the scarf under the leg.

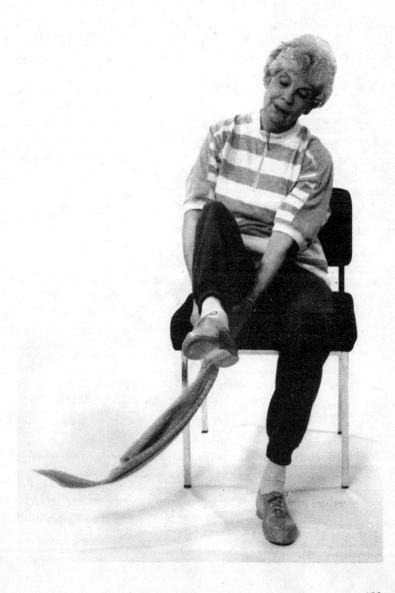

- Catch the scarf in the left hand, put right leg back on floor and lift the left leg then swing back the scarf under the left leg into the right hand, then swing it back under the leg into the right hand.

When you have finished with one leg, place it back on the floor, lift the other leg and work on that one.

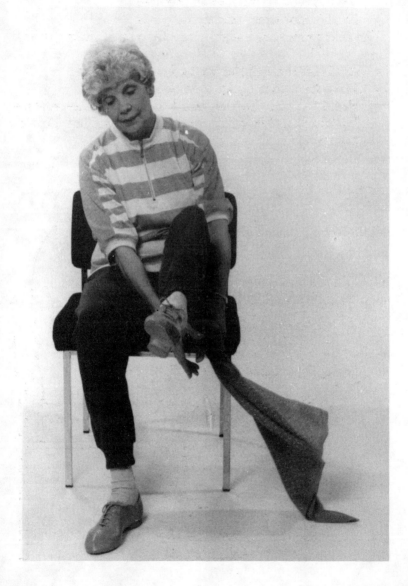

Working on your whole leg

You should be sitting upright in a chair again.

- Lift the right leg so that it is horizontal, with a straight knee.
- Point the toes up to the ceiling.
- Letting the chair take the weight of your leg, bend your leg and replace the foot on the floor.
- Do this four times on alternate legs.

The next exercise is a slightly tougher variation on the first one.

- Again lift the right leg so the knee is straight.
- Place the hands under the thigh for support.
- Point the toes down as much as possible, keeping the leg straight, then point them up to the ceiling. Do this four times.

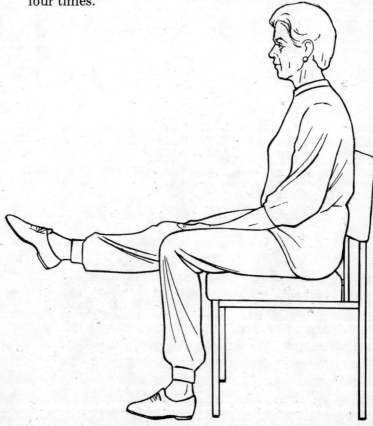

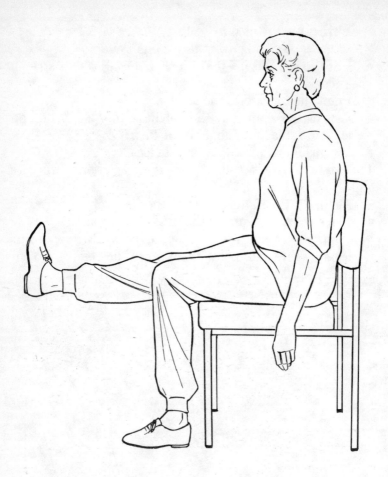

- Remove your hands from supporting your thigh and lift the right leg from the hip as far as you find comfortable. Do this three times.
- Replace the right foot gently on the floor.
- Repeat with the other leg.

If you do this exercise quickly and rhythmically you will find it less tiring than doing it slowly. And here's another variation, this time with your knee bent.

- Put your hands under your right thigh.
- Keeping your knee bent and relaxed, lift your right leg up with your hands and gently pull it towards your body without straining.

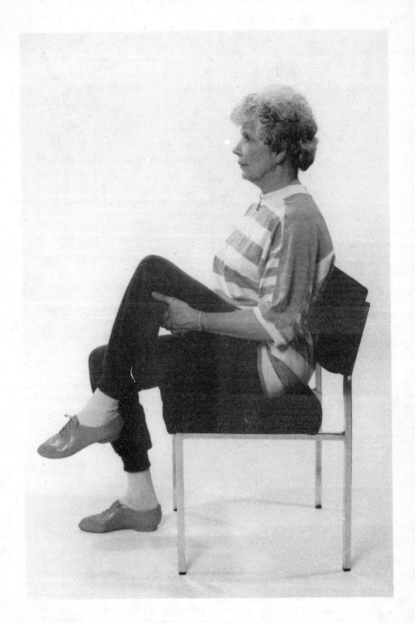

- Let your leg back down again and replace your foot on the floor.
- Repeat with the other leg.

Do the complete movement four times in all.

Walking your bottom
Again, you should be seated upright in a chair.
- Put your hands on either side of the seat of the chair —
  you will need them there to steady you.
- Now, with your feet remaining flat on the floor, walk
  your buttocks forwards four times and backwards four
  times, so you are back where you started.
- Repeat the movement once.

Keep the movements small, otherwise you'll 'walk' off the
front of the chair and land on the floor.

USEFUL INFORMATION

Ramblers' Association
1–5 Wandsworth Road
London SW18 2LJ
01-582 6878

Society of Chiropodists
53 Welbeck Street
London W1M 7HE
01-486 3381/4

Varicose Veins, Professor Harold Ellis, Macdonald
Optima/Positive Health Guides, £4.99

11
MENTAL
EXERCISE

As we get older our memory often starts to fail us. Nobody quite knows why this happens but one thing seems fairly certain — the brain, including the memory, is just like our muscles in that if we don't use it, it starts to weaken. If we think of our memory as needing exercise like a muscle, then we can think of ways of working on it.

Obviously, if the loss of memory is caused by a degenerative illness such as senile dementia, there is no cure (at the moment). However, for ordinary bad memories there are a few things we can do to try and improve them.

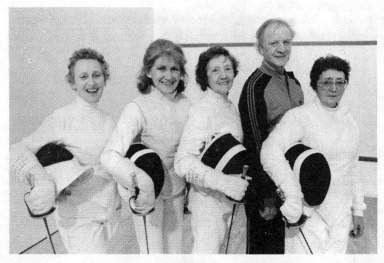

Above all — have fun!

USE YOUR BRAIN

Try learning something new every day. Memorise a phone number or learn a piece of poetry by heart and then test yourself on it. Get into the habit of trying to memorise something every day, however small.

If you have trouble remembering things such as a name or a number, try imagining it written up on a big sign or put to a piece of music that you like. Or try to make an amusing connection with the name. All these tricks make things easier to remember.

I play scrabble on my own. I helps to keep your mind active and also helps you to learn new words. I also play patience by myself. Again, it's a matter of keeping active. When you live alone you want your brain to keep going.

Helen, 67.

HELP YOUR MEMORY

Some researchers think that various vitamins and minerals can have an effect on the memory.

Vitamin B_5, in particular, other vitamins in the B complex, and vitamin C are thought to help, as is ginseng — available in health-food shops. Wheatgerm, spinach, bran, asparagus, mushrooms, fish, onions, oatmeal and chicken-liver are all thought to contain nutrients good for stimulating the memory, so try to include them in your diet.

Learning to relax can also help your ability to concentrate — try yoga to calm your mind. And if you have trouble remembering everyday things, get into the habit of keeping a diary and making lists. Keep a notebook handy wherever you go and write down thoughts as they occur to you.

Learning a basic exercise routine that you have to remember and concentrate on each time you do it can help to keep your memory working well.

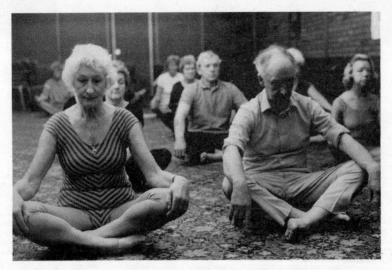

Practising yoga helps to calm your mind.

DRUGS AND YOUR MEMORY

If you are taking drugs on a regular basis, especially tranquillisers or sleeping pills, they can affect your memory. It
may be worth asking your doctor if you can reduce or even
stop your daily dose if it is having this effect, but don't
stop taking them without medical advice.

If you want extra help to stop taking tranquillisers,
contact Tranx (UK) Ltd.

MENTAL EXERCISE

Boredom kills — it's an old saying, but it's true. However
fit your body is, if your mind isn't kept active you won't be
at your best.

If you are able to get out and about you should be able
to find other people to chat to and activities to join in with.
Age Concern run local groups or can help set up one if
there aren't any in your area. And they can also advise
you on the availability of help with transport to and from
group meetings.

> I like playing cards. I enjoy the competition.
>
> *Kathleen*, 55.

Or you could try taking a day or evening class. Ask at your local adult education institute what classes are available locally. Your local library will also have details of clubs and activities available in your area.

Other organisations which run classes, courses and exams in various subjects include the University of the Third Age — this in particular specialises in courses for those that have retired — the Open University and the Workers' Educational Association (WEA). You often find that the WEA run local classes, with special rates for pensioners.

MENTAL EXERCISE AT HOME

If you don't feel up to joining a class or if you are housebound, you can still keep your brain ticking over. Try joining in with the quiz shows on television. If you don't know the answer, have a guess anyway. Do the competitions in magazines or in those free newspapers that come through the letterbox. You don't have to send in your entry — you've still had the benefit of exercising your mind.

Card and board games are an excellent way of keeping your brain active. There are chess, scrabble, domino and card clubs around, or you could get together with friends for a game on a regular basis. Don't forget that some card games you can play on your own.

READING

Or you could increase the amount or the range of reading you do. You don't have to rely on new books — there are many secondhand bookshops around, or see what you can find at your local jumble sales.

Most people are near a library, where you will find a wealth of reading material that you can borrow for nothing. And most libraries also serve as a noticeboard for organisations and information — there's no knowing what you might find out about there.

If your eyesight isn't what it used to be, you can make use of the large-print books that are widely available now — again, your local library will have a good range. And if you really can't see well enough to read at all, why not arrange to get audio cassettes of newspapers, magazine and books.

USEFUL INFORMATION

Age Concern England
60 Pitcairn Road
Mitcham
Surrey CR4 3LL
01-640 5431

Age Concern Wales
1 Park Grove
Cardiff CF1 3BJ
0222 371821/371556

Age Concern Scotland
33 Castle Street
Edinburgh EH2 3DN
031-225 5000

Age Concern Ireland
128 Great Victoria Street
Belfast BT2 7BG
0232 245729

University of the Third Age
6 Parkside Gardens
London SW19 5EY
Send a stamped addressed envelope if you want to find out about classes and groups in your area.

Open University
Enquiry Office
PO Box 71
Bucks MK7 6AA
0908 653212
The Open University run both degree courses and shorter courses, with course material being transmitted on TV and radio as well as local tutorials, meetings, etc., and summer schools. Write and find out more.

Workers' Educational Association
9 Upper Berkeley Street
London W1H 8BY
01-402 5608/9

Talking Newspaper Association UK (TNAUK)
90 High Street
Heathfield
East Sussex TN12 8JD
04352 6102
TNAUK supplies audio cassettes of newspapers and magazines.

Calibre
Aylesbury
Bucks HP20 1HV
0296 81211 or 0296 432339 (24 hours)
Calibre supply audio cassettes of books.

Tranx (UK) Ltd
25A Masons Avenue
Wealdstone
Harrow
Middlesex HA3 5AH
01-427 2065 or 01-427 2827 (24 hours)
Tranx will provide advice and information if you are trying to stop taking tranquillisers, or having problems with them.

Mensa
Bond House
St John's Square
Wolverhampton WV2 4AH
or
Freepost
Wolverhampton WV2 1BR

Royal National Institute for the Blind
224 Great Portland Street
London W1N 6AA
01-388 1266

Royal National Institute for the Deaf and the British Tinnitus Association
105 Gower Street
London WC1E 6AH
01-387 8033

British Association of the Hard of Hearing
7-11 Armstrong Road
London W3 7JL
01-743 1110

Disabled Living Foundation
380-84 Harrow Road
London W9 2HU
01-289 6111

More books from Optima

Acupuncture Michael Nightingale ISBN 0-356-12426-6,
£3.95

Answers to Asthma Dr Chris Sinclair ISBN
0-356-12435-5, £3.95

Answers to Migraine Dr Clifford Rose and Dr Paul Davies,
ISBN 0-356-12437-1, £3.95

Below the Belt Denise Winn, ISBN 0-356-12740-0, £3.95

Coping with Multiple Sclerosis Cynthia Benz, ISBN
0-356-12793-1, £5.99

Coping with Old Age Pat Blair, ISBN 0-356-12794-X,
£4.95 (December 1988)

Herbal Medicine Anne McIntyre, ISBN 0-356-12429-0,
£3.95

Menopause the Natural Way Dr Sadja Greenwood, ISBN
0-356-12561-0, £5.95

Private Parts: A Health Book for Men Yosh Taguchi,
ISBN 0-356-15556-0, £5.99

POSITIVE HEALTH GUIDES

Anxiety and Depression Professor Robert Priest, ISBN
0-356-14460-7, £5.99

Beat Heart Disease Risteard Mulcahy, ISBN
0-356-14464-X, £4.99

Caring for an Elderly Relative Dr Keith Thompson, ISBN
0-356-14465-8, £5.99

Cervical Smear Test Albert Singer FRCOG and Dr Anne Szarewski, ISBN 0-356-15065-8, £5.99

Diabetes: A Beyond Basics Guide Dr Rowan Hillson, ISBN 0-356-14545-0, £4.95

Healthy Heart Diet Book Professor Jim Mann and Roberta Longstaff, SRD, ISBN 0-356-14488-7, £5.99

High Blood Pressure Dr Eoin O'Brien and Professor Kevin O'Malley, ISBN 0-356-14489-5, £4.95

High-Fibre Cookbook Pamela Westland, ISBN 0-356-14490-9, £5.99

Menopause Dr Jean Coope, ISBN 0-356-14511-5, £5.99

Migraine and Headaches Dr Maria Wilkinson, ISBN 0-356-14496-8, £4.99

Overcoming Arthritis Dr Frank Dudley Hart, ISBN 0-356-14498-4, £4.99

Salt Free Diet Book Dr Graham MacGregor, ISBN 0-356-14503-4, £4.99

Stroke: A Practical Guide to Recovery Dr Richard Langton and Dr Derrick T Wade, ISBN 0-356-14454-2, £5.99